TROJAN
WORKOUT

MARTIJN BOS
with
MARTY GALLAGHER

TROJAN
WORKOUT

MARTIJN BOS
with
MARTY GALLAGHER

© Copyright 2018, Martijn Bos
A Dragon Door Publications, Inc. production
All rights under International and Pan-American Copyright conventions.
Published in the United States by: Dragon Door Publications, Inc.
5 East County Rd B, #3 • Little Canada, MN 55117
Tel: (651) 487-2180 • Fax: (651) 487-3954
Credit card orders: 1-800-899-5111 • Email: support@dragondoor.com • Website: www.dragondoor.com

ISBN-10: 1-942812-16-7   ISBN-13: 978-1-942812-16-6
This edition first published in January 2019
Printed in China

No part of this book may be reproduced in any form or by any means without the prior written consent of the Publisher, excepting brief quotes used in reviews.

BOOK DESIGN: Derek Brigham • www.dbrigham.com • bigd@dbrigham.com

PHOTOGRAPHY: Author photo and interior photos by Picture People.

DISCLAIMER: The authors and publisher of this material are not responsible in any manner whatsoever for any injury that may occur through following the instructions contained in this material. The activities, physical and otherwise, described herein for informational purposes only, may be too strenuous or dangerous for some people and the reader(s) should consult a physician before engaging in them. The content of this book is for informational and educational purposes only and should not be considered medical advice, diagnosis, or treatment. Readers should not disregard, or delay in obtaining, medical advice for any medical condition they may have, and should seek the assistance of their health care professionals for any such conditions because of information contained within this publication.

— TABLE OF CONTENTS —

FOREWORD
AUTHOR'S NOTE
PART 1 1
Martial Roots 1
Adolescent Fight Training 6
Korps Commando Troepen (KCT) 11
Sport Academy, MMA and a Bolt of Martial Lightning 14
Fighters Fight 17
Krav Maga 19
Practical Fitness Training 22
Reality Check 25
High School Hell 26
Real World Workshop 29
My 15 Minutes of Fame 30
Secondary School Purgatory and Taking the Plunge 36
Formulating Philosophies 37
Hogeschool 39
Real Life Experience 42
Transitioning 43
Kettlebell Thunderbolt 46
The Right Tool at the Right Time for the Right Man: Slow Power is NoPpower 47
The Emperor has no clothes 49
The Radical Experiment: the Trojan Workout Challenge 52
Sandy 57
Monumental Quest 64
Skill Testing 67
The Fast 71
Post-certification De-brief 73

PART 2 TROJAN WORKOUT 75
Conceptual Beginnings 75
Philosophic Underpinnings 77
The Psychology of the True Trojan 78
Compete with Yourself! Learn to Love the Process! 80
Coping with Fatigue 81
Put in the Work 82
The Mental Effort Intensity Scale (MEIS) 84
Keep a Positive Mental Attitude (PMA) 86
The Trojan Workout versus running 87
The Trojan Workout versus High Intensity Training (HIT) 89
The Sea Squirt 90
Trojan Workout Goal Setting 91

PART 3 93
Your First Trojan Workout… 93
Group Lessons 97
Tools of a Trojan 98
Isometric Holds: The Trojan Pose 101
Exercises 104
Trojan Sets 133
Training Tips When Training at Home (No Group Session) 134
Trojan Workout for Self Defense 134
Krav Maga in Motion 137

FOREWORD
By Avi Moyal

New fitness trends seem to emerge every other day—and most of them it seems to me have originated in Hong Kong or New York. So I was extremely surprised by Dutch-born Martijn Bos's ***Trojan Workout*** which contains a new and refreshing approach towards fitness, along with deep insights into a subject that is so dear to me: Martial Arts.

Well written, deeply researched and professionally produced, Trojan Workout conveys a knowledge that is backed up by Martijn's practical life experience. Trojan Workout highlights the physical, cognitive and mental training behind the combat techniques and tactics essential to a professional fighter as well as to anyone in a real life-threatening situation.

The "Trojan Workout" principles are great for those who seek fitness and strength, integrated with realistic experience, and these are the motifs I was glad to find in this book.

It is also a wonderful way to complete the knowledge of IKMF Krav Maga, as it was founded by Imi and continues to grow and improve through the creative and gifted minds of this new generation.

Avi Moyal
Master in Krav Maga, Head instructor IKMF

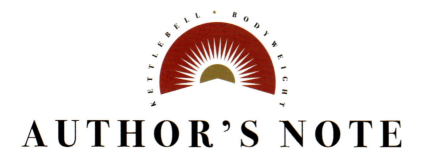

AUTHOR'S NOTE

Voor Lucy en Jonas. Ik hou van jullie tot het einde van de ruimte en terug

Could Trojan Workout change the world? That's a bold proposition indeed...

Well, it changed my world—dramatically—and I believe it can change yours too. In fact, *anybody* who applies themselves with the proper intensity can get and feel stronger, using the Trojan Workout principles.

It's not that you always have to be strong, but the feeling of strength is more important than winning or losing in life. And strength is already within you. You just need to earn it by giving it attention. I hope my book empowers you to have the life you want and that you feel strong, confident and joyful.

From an early age I've always had the desire to help others. I guess my mother showed me how. Today I own Trainingscentrum Helena where me and my team of instructors help improve people's physical and mental strength. We teach Krav Maga, Trojan Workout and mental power principles. My other company Martijn Bos Academy helps high performers to reach their full potential. What I see when I'm coaching is that most of them also have a desire to help others. Born out of their personal struggle comes an urge to empower other people with the lessons they have learned.

When I decided to write this book, I had the same objective. I want to share how any-body, I mean ANYBODY can live up to their full potential.

This book has three parts:

The first part is about my personal story—how I've grown from my early challenges and what my road has been so far. By sharing my story, I hope you can see that I'm not a privileged or talented person that got my success as a gift. I've struggled, fought and failed on many occasions. What made me successful was that I never gave up. I've made a lot of mistakes, but losing hope was never one of them. I kept trying, I kept showing up. Learning from something is always an option and you should always stay positive; don't freeze, keep moving. Never give up.

If you would step away from the idea that you need to gain strength and see that growing stronger is our natural birthright, you will discover that it's easier to continue showing up for your workout. Instead of putting heavy demands on yourself, just pay attention to the potential that is already within you and identify the things that are making you weak. You only compete with yourself. Strength is already within us all. You just need to put in the effort of getting to use it. You need to earn it, but it's already yours.

In part 2, you will find the mental power principles that will help you to earn your strength. I learned these principles within Krav Maga and have applied them to Trojan Workout. These principles are universal and applicable in multiple situations. Not just in fitness, but in life. Keep them front and center.

Part 3 is all about learning the Trojan Workout. Make Trojan Workout part of your life—it will empower you, improve your health and give you a sharper mind and stronger body. Let Trojan Workout be part of your daily routine and reward yourself with an easy, highly effective way of training that you can do for the rest of your life.

Nobody gets to the finish alone. A special thanks to:

Papa, for all that you have given me
Suzanne, for your love, support, care and acceptance
Ben Hulskamp, your teaching changed my life and showed me my personal strength
John Du Cane, for the opportunity to share my story
Marty Gallagher, for making sure my readers understand what I want to tell them

My instructors working at Trainingscentrum Helena and all my students that let me practice my ideas, principles and training on them. Without you, Trojan Workout would still be just an idea.

All the people that helped me bring my book to fruition, including; Avi Moyal, Dr. Mark Atkinson, Mylaissa van Gool, Positivity Branding, Marloes Coenen, Lucia Rijker, Picture People Amstelveen, Nick Kailola.

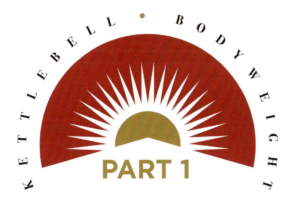

PART 1

MARTIAL ROOTS

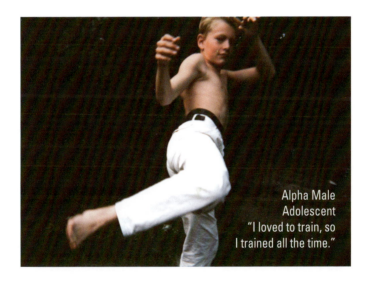

Alpha Male Adolescent
"I loved to train, so I trained all the time."

I was born and raised in Alphen aan den Rijn. Alphen on the Rhine is located in the western Netherlands, in the province of South Holland between Leiden and Utrecht. My hometown is situated on the banks of the river Oude Rijn.

Alphen on the Rhine has a population of around 100,000 people and is in what is called the 'Green Heart' of the Netherlands. I was born and raised there.

My father was a teacher and my mother was a homemaker. Both my mother and father were deeply religious, strict Christians that became even more strict and more devout when my mother was diagnosed with cancer. I was two years old. The cancer took twelve years to kill my mother. It devastated our family, tearing it apart on every level. Financially, the illness decimated our standard of living. Emotionally, it destroyed my father. He became distant as he dealt with my mother's death in his own way.

After years of battling cancer, with some ups and a lot of downs, my mother died. I was 14. I dealt with my mother's passing in my own way. It imprinted me. Her sickness, her struggle, her death and its aftermath remain the single most devastating thing that has ever happened to me. Children subjected to trauma are often deeply affected and become emotionally scarred. My mother's valiant struggle, how she dealt with death and dying, formed the foundation of what and who I am today. Struggle in the face of overwhelming odds and death are to me, the most noble of undertakings. Her gallantry in the face of death inspired me and provided me a character benchmark.

My mother's name was Helena, as in Helena of Troy. I named my company Trainingscentrum Helena as a tribute to her. The strength of character my mother exhibited inspires me to this day. She spent all the last years of her life battling cancer—yet her greatest joy during that period was helping others.

Helena walked through life courageously. My strongest impressions of her were how she continually sought ways to become stronger, mentally and physically. She had every reason to complain and never did. Instead she focused on her diet and lifestyle. Despite all the hospital visits and chemotherapy treatments, Helena always showed strength.

Helena always managed to bring out the best in herself and in others. With her infinite optimism and strong life force, she was an inspiration to many. She accepted her suffering and focused on how she could improve her health and how she could help others. Offering help was her calling. Friends and family always came to her for advice.

She motivated my father to continue studying. She stimulated me to do my best at school and did not accept it when I did half work. I developed my sense of giving and community from her example. She selflessly sought to help others. That ideal motivates me to this day.

How can I, a professional martial artist, help others? Allow everyone the ability to feel safe. Enable people to become stronger, physically and psychologically. How can I help others succeed?

I have devised a system of self-defense and fitness that enables anyone at any level to improve. Everyone, regardless their level of fitness or unfitness, can and will grow stronger, physically and psychologically, by routinely practicing the Trojan workout.

I stress the melding of mental with physical. The goal is to train both the physiological and the psychological. Build a better stronger body and simultaneously build a better stronger mind. The Trojan workout ingrains life skills—stressing focus, awareness, goal attainment and the clichéd (yet factually accurate) idea of improving self-esteem. It might sound trite, but it is important to feel good about who and what you are.

Anyone can exhibit courage and class when things are going well and everyone is prosperous and happy—the true test is, who can show courage and strength when things are going badly? My entire approach is based on the idea of creating skills that can be called on and used during the most trying of times and most dangerous of situations.

The goal of the Trojan Workout is to overcome resistance, to stand strong in training and to stand strong in life. To be effective on a variety of levels requires a melding of the physical and the mental. Anyone at any level can make astounding progress, mentally and physically, following the precepts of the Trojan workout. Everyone, everywhere has a wish to be strong and safe. Our training makes a person strong—and by radically improving strength we make a person safer.

I founded Trainingscentrum Helena in 2005. I had a mission: first and foremost, I wanted Trainingscentrum Helena to be more than just a regular gym. I dreamed of a training center where people would go to work on both their physical and mental strength. I found this blending of physical and mental in the principles of Krav Maga. I later used the same principles as the foundation for the Trojan Workout.

My training programs make people stronger. "Stand strong in your shoes!"

As a child, I had to deal with heavy experiences that had a big impact on me. My mother was dying and that hung over me like a dark cloud. I was bullied at school and I was bullied in the neighborhood where I lived. I was a skinny, sullen, depressed kid, with no real friends. Being quiet and alone, I was always a favorite target for school bullies.

I had to run home from school every day as fast as I could so as not to be caught and given "a strong beating." I felt unsafe and insecure. I suspect the high pain tolerance I have today is a result of being on the receiving end of so many punches and kicks from much larger and more powerful opponents.

I had my first introduction to martial arts watching Bruce Lee movies. Here was a small, skinny guy like me that had turned himself into a fighting machine. As a young boy, I would get so enthused watching Bruce Lee that I would leap up to imitate Lee's movie techniques. After watching his movies, I would practice my Bruce Lee imitation moves on imaginary opponents for hours at a time.

I developed the strong imagination that is common to lonely children. In my mind's eye, I would use my Kung Fu to defeat much larger and more formidable imaginary opponents. These mental images became so strong that, for me, it became an alternate reality. While my reality was a home life that was bleak, poor and depressing, by contrast my imaginary Kung Fu world was electric and exciting with heroes (me) and villains to be vanquished.

This early martial imaging would serve me well for the rest of my life. Mental recalibration, focus, concentration, using the power of the Mind to improve performance and overcome adversity and obstacles had their beginnings with my intense visualizations as a young boy.

My mother's cancer was hard for my father. During my mother's illness, my dad became more withdrawn as she succumbed. He disliked my passion for martial arts. I craved his approval. His grief twisted his perceptions. I became a 'latch-key kid' without much adult supervision. With my mother dead and my father always away from home, I felt non-stop loneliness. I quit school and I suddenly had a lot of time on my hands. As the old saying goes, "Idle time is the Devil's workshop."

In the months before my mother's death, I had encountered an instructor who schooled me on the karate basics: stance, movement fore and aft, how to make a fist, how to throw a punch; it was an odd time and this was an odd fellow.

Yes, he was knowledgeable insofar as the basics. He showed me sound techniques—but it seemed to me that he wanted to build a cult around himself. He demanded obedience that went way outside the role of student and teacher. He was always testing me. His demands were arbitrary and unreasonable.

I stopped training with him when he told me that attending my mother's funeral was no excuse for missing a training session with him. I walked out on him that day and never saw his face again. His horrible behavior shaped my approach towards the relationship I nowadays have with my own students. I treat my students with the respect and professionalism that I deserved and that they deserve.

After ditching the karate instructor, I took what knowledge I'd accumulated and began training by myself. I discovered that I was a self-motivator. Whereas for most students their wild and uncontrollable mind is their worst enemy, for me, my mind was my best friend. I loved to train, so I trained all the time. The solo training approach suited me just fine.

I was 16 years old. I lived at home and trained from dawn to dusk. I became a martial monk. My every waking hour was spent either training or thinking about training.

My Mind became my best friend. I focused my life and my very existence on improving my skillset as a fighter. When you train alone, it is hard to be objective about your own progress. You think you are progressing—but are you? I strove for increases in performance in the various drills. I could always train harder and more often, I could train longer. I would set new push up goals, strive for new chin up records.

All of which was great from a "better body" perspective—but was I improving as a fighter? There needs to be real world applicability. Was I a gym trainer or a fighter? At my core, I knew that I was a fighter and I felt the need to fight!

There needs to be something buried in a person's psychological makeup that makes them enthusiastic about real combat with another human. Very few people are hardwired to be fighters. There are a lot of people that love the idea of being a fighter—but that is different than someone who truly, deeply enjoys and looks forward to hitting another human in the face and just as importantly (more so?) has a naturally high pain tolerance and persistence that allows them to shrug off getting smashed in the face with a fist or kick. I decided I needed to test myself and fight.

ADOLESCENT FIGHT TRAINING

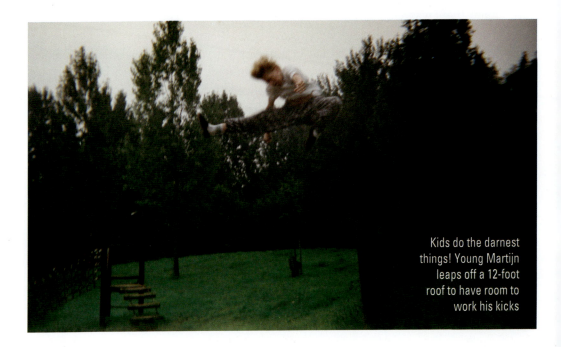

Kids do the darnest things! Young Martijn leaps off a 12-foot roof to have room to work his kicks

As a youngster, I sought to imitate the choreographed punches and kicks that my movie heroes used to dispatch opponents. I was particularly taken with the acrobatic high kicks and sought to replicate them. I must have practiced 10,000 high kicks. Like anything else, practice makes perfect and all those leaping kicks I performed as a kid actually laid a terrific foundation for my future fight efforts.

As a pretend martial arts expert imitating my heroes, I ran, leapt, spun, rolled and mastered every type and kind of jumping kick. Like any other teen fighter, I wanted to masterfully perform incredible kicks, the flashier and more complex the better!

Jean Claude Van Damme and Bruce Lee were my role models. I was transfixed by the athletic abilities these two men exhibited. I watched all their movies and the instant I saw a new move I would leap up and immediately began imitating it. I became a sponge for their incredible leg work. They exhibited precision, power and grace. To this day, no one has done what they did better.

I discovered that the longer you were airborne the more elaborate your kicks could be. So very early on I sought ways in which to increase my hang time. How do you create more time airborne? Jump off something elevated, a table, box, a diving board or a roof. I leapt off a lot of roofs. Almost as important as learning the kicks was learning how to land.

When you leap off a roof, you have to learn how to fall and roll and absorb the ground impact, otherwise your roof-leaping career will be cut short by catastrophic injury. All my martial art leaping, running, jumping, landing was extremely beneficial. I was unwittingly performing foundational Parkour training before Parkour was invented.

The other way to increase hang time, I reasoned was to find a way to get way stronger legs, powerhouse legs that allow a fighter to jump higher. The higher a fighter can leap, the longer his hang time. I was always practicing jumping kicks. Even as a boy I instinctively and intuitively sought ways in which to improve.

Over time I developed a training template. Rather than just being a wild boy, doing whatever came into his feral mind at that instant, I developed a very rudimentary and extremely basic daily training regimen, a regular schedule of formalized training. My strategy combined a formalized series of jumping and leaping that I would combine with lightning-fast strike skills. I worked up an entire repertoire. I would perform a leaping kick and upon landing immediately go into rapid-fire shadow boxing and kicking. It looked cool and made me feel like a movie hero. Some of my regular boy/teen protocols included...

- Leaping off a table or ledge — extra height creates more hang time
- Leaping from the ground — consciously seek to improve vertical leap
- Sprint, leap and kick — turning horizontal speed into vertical ascent
- Jumping kick drill — done sequentially at a fast, even pace
- Jumping kicks sets — 10-30 kata reps without rest
- Rest between sets — vary the rest periods
- My teen mantra — the more you leap and kick, the better at it you become

Another drill I invented was lying down flat on the ground, then leaping up as fast as I could and once on my feet I would commence a rapid-fire punch/kick attack. I would lie on the ground in many different poses, differing variations, i.e. lying face down, lying on my back, lying on my side, leaning on my hands, curled up, from the push-up position... I would leap upward as fast as humanly possible. This was a functional self-defense burpee. Done for long sequences, these 'get-ups' not only built strength and stamina, they also improved agility and sharpened reflexes.

They say necessity is the mother of invention and this is also true in martial arts. My 'ground get-up' drills were created at a time I was being roughed up by older, larger boys. I found myself on the ground continually with some oversized bully sitting or lying atop me, trying to hit me and certainly squishing me. These scramble-drills had me bouncing back up the instant I got knocked to the ground. This tactic was born out of necessity and only years later did I discover that this was an advanced and quite sophisticated fighting tactic.

Today I still do (weight-bearing) variations and versions of these same scramble drills. Nowadays when I come up off the ground, I am performing a Turkish get-up with a heavy kettlebell in my hand. The strategy is the same. In 2017 I use kettlebells to amplify the effort and the results. One of my favorite drills in 2017 was first conceived in 1997. How cool is that.

Very early on I began linking isometric (or grind tension) exercise with high velocity speed work. The contrasting combination, all-out static strength immediately followed by lightning fast movement, creates unique and outstanding physiological results.

One repeating theme that I use to this day had its genesis when I was a teenager. The protocol is to link exercises together, do them one after another, without rest.

Another repeating theme I use to this day: alternate isometric, isotonic or grind exercises are followed *instantaneously* by an explosive exercise. Alternate grind movements with explosive movements; high tension exercise followed by an explosive exercise.

Long exercise chains should be constructed using contrasting intensities. One illustrative example: perform a Turkish Get-up with a heavy kettlebell. Upon completion immediately begin a series of high velocity kicks and punches. Continue until lactic acid buildup occurs. Fight through the burn. After lactic acid buildup shuts down the ability to punch or kick, commence a third exercise, a series of "leg only" plyometric-type leaps, bounds and jumps. Now loop back around to an isometric exercise to repeat the three-exercise sequence.

On every series of exercises, on every exercise, seek to drive deeper into the lactic acid pain zone. Over time and with repeated practice, the ability to linger longer in the lactic acid pain zone improves. The perfect exercise should tax the athlete physically and psychologically. Learn how to pivot from extreme isometric-type exertion into instantaneous explosiveness. Over time, longer exercise chains of exercises can be linked. Time spent in the lactic acid fatigue zone is time well spent.

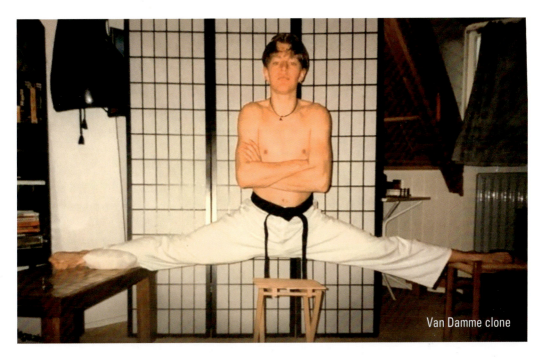

Van Damme clone

I entered the Dutch Open National karate championship at the age of 16 without any formal karate background. Just through training on my own, I made it to the semifinals. I lost a curious decision to a man 20 years older and 35 pounds heavier than me. I found out a lot about myself in that period. I discovered that my solo path, what I had been doing, was of real benefit. I also discovered that some drills I had been doing were a complete waste of time. After the championship I took up Thai Boxing and Muay Thai. I devoted more time to Karate.

The more I trained, the more I wanted to learn. I improved with every fight. I learned I had a high tolerance for pain—perhaps a result of being assaulted by bullies repeatedly as a youngster. I seemed to be able to take a punch and apparently, had the opposite of the glass jaw. I could take a licking and keep on ticking.

Fighting was exhilarating and electric. Anything could happen and I never felt more alive and complete than when I was circling an opponent intent on knocking me unconscious and choosing not to back down. I did not know it at the time, but my brain seemed to be hardwired for fighting. I reacted instinctually and intuitively—and usually correctly—in live combat.

Without thinking about it, I was reacting correctly when dealing with an incoming punch or kick. Without thinking about it, I would see an offensive opening and again, without thought would seize the opportunity to throw the right counter-blow from the right angle.

Was my savant-like martial reaction time a result of my immersion in training? Was it some sort of genetic gift—like being born with a beautiful singing voice or being born 7-foot tall? Skills can be improved upon with more training and better training, whereas genetic gifts are birthed, fully formed and complete.

By age 19 I had attained my full height, 6-foot, and weighed a light and lean 155 pounds. I started to think about my next move and how I could continue to improve myself. I was looking for a physical challenge that could keep me on my toes.

I joined the Army. I wanted to become a commando. I wanted to get out of Alphen. I wanted to become a professional warrior.

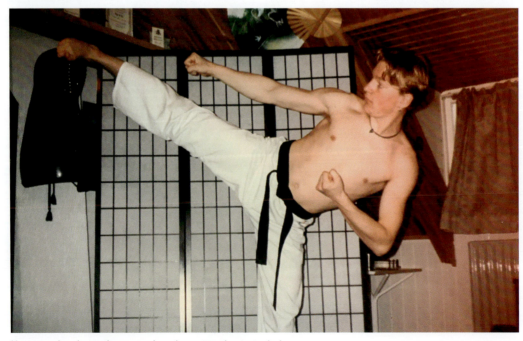

Young and serious: always paying close attention to technique

KORPS COMMANDO TROEPEN (KCT)

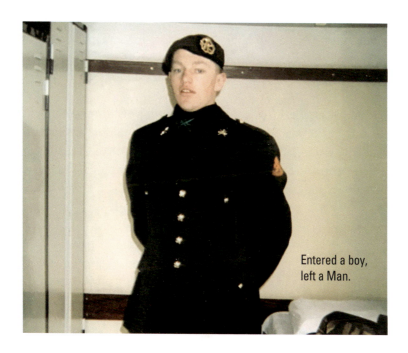

Entered a boy, left a Man.

The Korps Commandotroepen (KCT) is the Special Forces of the Royal Dutch Army. The KCT is the elite of the elite and is deployable anywhere in the world under any circumstance. The KCT conducts a full spectrum of special operations missions. Characterized by its signature green beret, the KCT accepts applications from both active army personnel (infantry) and civilians.

In 1998 I was 19 years old and in tiptop physical and mental shape. I made the decision that I wanted to become a green beret, a member of the KCT, a commando, a professional warrior. I was a good civilian candidate. I could certainly fight, and I was in excellent physical condition. I was thin and light, 155 pounds on a six-foot frame. Trying out for the KCT made perfect sense.

Joining the army was a way out of my claustrophobic existence. Hometown life was grinding me down. In some ways, I had worked my whole life immersed in fighting, conflict and combat. While I could have used more muscle, my endurance, reflexes, speed and agility were peaked and fine-tuned. Though I was only 19, I already had a decade of fight training under my gi belt.

I had a secret weapon: my persistence. I was used to physical and psychological pain. I got my persistence and my psychological strength from my mother. I knew from fighting that I had a capacity to shrug off pain and keep going. I knew how to take a prolonged beating. Psychologically, my stressed-out home life and low-income living gave me a frame of reference. I had a streak of desperation, lacking in nice boys from safe comfortable homes. I took great pride in my ability to get knocked down and stand right back up.

I was also a bright youngster. I was not a brainless thug: my intense study of the martial arts turned me into a facile reader. I had an inquisitive mind and a tough upbringing. If any civilians made the KCTs, I thought I would be a civilian with a real chance. Above all else, I truly felt that I was a warrior. And while I might fail, I would not quit—ever. I joined the army and immediately signed up for KCT tryouts. I was given a date, place and time to report.

To be considered for the KCT, all civilian and military candidates had to participate in a three-day tryout that tested physical and mental stamina. Called Phase Zero, psychologists made a profile of each participant. Various demanding physical skills were tested, participants were graded on strength and stamina. For experienced military, the "wash-out" rate for Phase Zero was 70-80%. The wash-out rate was over 85% for civilians.

The civilian candidates that pass Phase Zero are sent to General Commando Military school. This phase is rough: a 17-week course in basic military skills and endless drills. Civilian candidates that get through General Commando Military School now join the military candidates and train together for four weeks. Most of this phase is done outside of Roosendaal, in the Belgian highlands and mountains.

The dismissal rate is high during this brutal four-week phase. Those that make it are eligible to attend Elementary Commando Education school. For the next fourteen weeks soldiers are put through the most grueling and demanding drills imaginable. The final week, week 14, is called Hell Week. For seven straight days and nights soldiers are subjected to unrelenting, continuous activity, including escape and evasion, forced marches, speed marches and sleep deprivation. Hell Week concludes with a forced march carrying a full load to the KCT headquarters. The remaining candidates are awarded the Green Beret.

Heading into the selection process, I was the youngest, smallest and thinnest candidate. Keep in mind that over 70% of hardened professional military men fail to make the KCTs. The percentage of civilians that make the cut was even smaller. Physically, I was unimposing. The grizzled military men were dismissive of me, the skinny kid civilian trying to become a KCT. There derisive laughter fueled my internal fire. They might be bigger and stronger, but I could outlast them.

I took great pleasure watching my tormentors fall to the wayside as the KCT selection process unfolded. Yet here I stood, eight weeks in, feeling really good about my chances. I had coped with every drill, mission and task, no matter how grueling, demanding or never-ending. There was a lot of exposure to the elements. It became more and more apparent to me and to the other KCT candidates that I was built to take it. I could keep putting one foot in front of the other, long past the point of utter and complete physical exhaustion. My willpower was extraordinary. I had an ability to endure. This trait is born in the mind.

During commando training we were allowed to go home on weekends. My father did not understand why I was doing what I was doing. He could not fathom why I would subject myself to this brutal training. Interestingly, despite his reservations, he took great care of me. He did my laundry, prepared my food and let me sleep as much as I needed—which was a lot. I am still grateful for his support during this incredibly demanding period. I could not have done it without him.

My quest to win the green beret was undone by an injury that occurred during a critical point in the selection process, just before Hell week. I was well on my way to being one of the youngest men ever to wear the Green Beret—but just when the goal was in my grasp, it was snatched away.

I was extremely grateful and flattered when my army commanders told me that in view of how well I had done and how far along I had gotten in the selection process, I would be allowed to try out for the Elementary Commando school once again.

To make a long story short, six weeks into my second try-out, I shattered my right foot in another training mishap. I walked for more than 15 kilometers with a broken foot while carrying a 20kg backpack.

My young mind was blown, my commando dreams were as shattered as my foot. My military career was over–and all inside of two years. Time to regroup, reflect and recalibrate.

SPORT ACADEMY, MMA AND A BOLT OF MARTIAL LIGHTNING

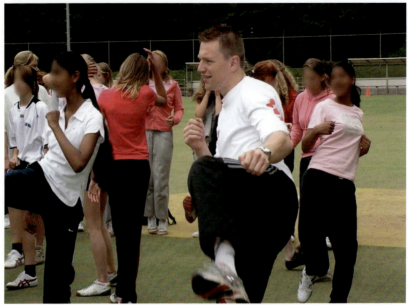

Sport Academy self-defense class: trying to suppress a smirk

By age 21, my military career was over. Two major injuries, each occurring at the most inopportune time, ended my life as a professional soldier. The most frustrating aspect of this phase of my life was that I really felt I was destined to be a commando. If I had somehow avoided the knee and foot injuries, there is zero doubt in my mind that I would have won my Green Beret. I don't quit. There is no doubt in my mind that I would have made an excellent soldier.

Physically and psychologically, I discovered that I was extremely well-suited for the commando lifestyle. I had certain intangible attributes that made me perfectly suited for elite military. Sure, I had the necessary physical skills, I was lean, fit, strong for my size and extremely agile and athletic. I could fight like a demon and run like the wind—but so could

Commando Troepen *all* the candidates are fit, fast, strong, lean and athletic. With a 90% fail rate, very few win the Green Beret.

I was skinny compared to all the muscled-up, tattooed giants that tried out when I did. If an outsider were to have viewed my tryout group for Korps on day one, I would have been the most physically unimposing of all the new recruits and the guy everyone would have picked as most likely to fail. Physiologically I was small. Psychologically I was a muscled-up, tattooed giant. When it came to the psychological aspects needed to succeed, my ability to endure set me apart and enabled me to outlast bigger, stronger, faster men.

The human body can be built up with expert training and consistency. Improving psychically, psychologically, by comparison, is far more difficult. The ability to endure, to persevere, to outlast, is something radically different, purely a psychological trait. My strongest attribute was my Mind—which made my exit from the military even more devastating. I was so certain that I had what it took to become a commando that I had not even considered any other career possibilities. Now I was injured and discharged and unsure of my next step.

The good news was that for the first time in my life I had a little bit of money. I was well compensated while in the military. Since I neither smoked, drank or had any serious romantic interests, I had saved most of my money. I did quite a lot of reflecting and came to two decisions: I wanted to become a fitness professional and I wanted to go to college, to University. I began researching Sport Academies.

When I came across Haagse Hogeschool located in The Hague, I became excited, really excited; if I could make the leap and land on my feet, if I could make the transition, I would be going from the maleness, the austereness and sparseness of commando life to the polar opposite: university life in one of the world's premier cities. My life would be full of possibilities, full of excitement, I could aspire to a new, higher level of training and meet beautiful women. What a cool possibility. My depression melted. I would embark on a brand new and completely different life path.

I enrolled in the academy and found a small room to rent. It was on an upper floor close to the University, a dormitory situation that I found exciting. The academy curriculum had two parts, physical and academic. The physical part consisted of classes in rhythmic and musical dance, self-defense, gymnastics, track and field and "game playing," soccer, tennis, baseball, etc. The academic classes were hard science: anatomy, physiology, didactics, kinesiology, nutrition and health. The classes were no joke.

While I had an advantage insofar as the athletic aspects of sport academy, the classwork and homework were quite intense. I had to apply myself. I learned a lot. Sport academy provided me with a knowledge base I use to this day. I was forced to learn about things that I never would have pursued on my own. The human body is an amazingly complicated and complex machine. My classes in anatomy and didactics taught me the function and relationship the mind and body have to one another.

I was taught to think from a scientific perspective. Scientists need to adopt an appropriate dispassionate attitude, using result-oriented empiricism to formulate a thesis. I would never have studied nutrition in the in-depth way University required. The broad array of topics and subjects allowed me to introduce science into my own training. The knowledge I was acquiring enabled me to take my physique and performance to the next level.

The first-year students like myself were younger than me and mostly came from nice homes and comfortable backgrounds. I was different. Being in top shape at a sports academy didn't hurt my popularity. I found that I could talk with the other students and the professors and we had a lot to talk about. I opened up and engaged people. I suppose I was considered a bit different, compared to my urban and suburban classmates.

My body and condition spoke volumes: I exemplified much of what was being taught and I already had what others sought: a fit, lean, functional body. I had a gravitas because I was an ex-commando and a fighter in tiptop shape. My fellow students had a lot of questions as to how I got that way. My transition from military to college was complete. I really liked this new life and began a whole new chapter in my life.

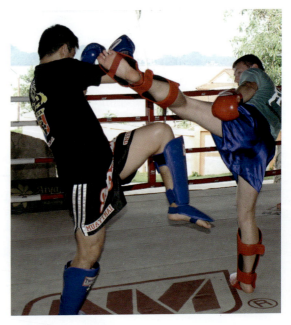

I recommenced my Muay Thai training. I was no longer in a small town. This was the big city and elite fight gyms were everywhere. In addition to attending classes, socializing with new friends, homework and study, I would travel across town and train for two hours 3-4 times a week. I did insane conditioning drills and lots of sparring. Physically, I was no longer skinny and underweight. I was weighing a ripped 180 pounds. I was in shape. I could hit hard, take a punch and could do cardio for days.

Muay Thai training: when not training, thinking about training

FIGHTERS FIGHT

I had watched with great interest the emerging Mixed Martial Arts format. The Ultimate Fighting Championship and Pride showcased the different fight schools as they battled one another for superiority. I was extremely impressed with the Brazilian ground fighters. They were a martial revelation. My background did not have any ground work, all my training had been in striking. The UFC and Pride opened an entire new universe of martial arts possibilities.

At some point my martial goal shifted. I no longer wanted to be "just" a striker, locked into one style, I wanted to become an MMA fighter. MMA training was opening my eyes and expanding my skills. I found I had a knack for grappling. Unlike a lot of natural strikers, I was extremely comfortable with ground fighting. I loved the chess match nature of grappling: move, countermove, counter-move to the counter-move. I was hungry to learn the innumerable submission techniques and when to clamp them on. I immersed myself in MMA, realizing that it was unquestionably the highest form of *sport* fighting.

My plan was to bring my MMA skill levels up to match my conditioning and toughness. I worked on seamless transitions, learning how to flow from one discipline to another, learning and then selecting the appropriate technique from jujitsu, karate, Muay Thai, sambo, wrestling, western boxing, I would select the technique as the situation dictated. I schooled myself on all the component parts; I just needed more mat time and lots of sparing sessions with top fighters. I learned to use all kinds and types of skills. I had all the unassembled puzzle pieces and I was learning how to put them together spontaneously and correctly.

At the highest level, fighting styles link. The transitions need to flow, fluidity is the whole game. Whereas once I sought to master all the old-school scripted and choreographed moves (the restrictions required when fighting within one style) I now wanted to be free of the "rules" associated with any one style.

Free form fighting needs flow. For me, the idea of transition flow inspired me. I developed a pro fighters appreciation for angles and subtleties. It was not a question of if I was going to become an MMA fighter, it was only a matter of when. It was a forgone conclusion that at some point in the not-too-distant future I would commence fighting on the MMA pro circuit.

In my second year at the University a bolt of martial lightning hit me and changed my life. The event was simple, mundane and average, I just happened to be watching TV one weekend afternoon (not something I do a lot of) and as I was flipping through the channels I came across a show on the Eurosport channel. Bored, I decided to watch. The show had a 15-minute segment on a "powerful new combat fighting art" called Krav Maga. The TV show related that Krav Maga was not sport fighting, rather an idiosyncratic self-defense system developed by the Israel special forces. I was instantly hypnotized.

What I saw on TV was a man, a Krav Maga master, fending off an incredible variety of attacks and then countering with some of the most ruthless counter-offensive blows I had ever seen. Knife attacks ended with the attacker being disarmed from his blade; multiple assailants were dispatched in rapid succession. Clubs and guns were neutralized and instantly turned on the assailant. I came up out of my chair. This was violence cubed—but counter-violence as opposed to offensive violence.

The Krav Maga defender, I later learned, was taught to "instinctively" create a response; maintain whatever space was needed to neutralize an attacker's attack. If the attacker cannot get close enough to land a death blow, the defender is safe and has time for prevention measures or to respond with a neutralizing counter-blow. And the responses were devastating. For me, the highlight of the segment was the Krav Maga expert's use of the groin kick.

In several instances, he used a smashing groin kick to instantly halt an attack. In the most extreme instance, during a one-on-one clinch, the Krav Maga expert fired four hard kicks, each landing on the attacker's private parts with the precision of a nuclear-tipped cruise missile. I remember thinking, *"Damn!* How simple can it be! I must learn THIS!"

In contrast to MMA, in the street or on the battlefield there are no referees, no rules, no rounds, no time outs and no tapping out and there are no weight classes. There are no weapons allowed in MMA. The illegal moves of sport fighting become the *best* moves for street fighting—what better offensive move than illegal ones that no one practices? Sport fighters never practice countermoves to illegal moves because there is no need.

As a scared and bullied preteen, I was a physical weakling that did not know how to stand up for myself. How could I? The martial movies were invaluable for sparking my initial interest. Karate competition provided the gateway from fantasy to reality. The military added the extreme conditioning so critical for fighting and MMA was the crown jewel of sport fighting—but what is beyond sport fighting?

KRAV MAGA

Krav Maga was the gateway from sport fighting to street fighting, from athletic contest to life and death. Once I saw Krav Maga in action, it spurred me to learn the philosophy behind Krav Maga. I declared my allegiance. I believed in the same things. In my heart of hearts, in my innermost martial soul, I am all about *preventing* a fight. I am not looking for a fight to win.

Being a great sport fighter no doubt helps at being a better combat fighter—but ultimately, sport and combat are two radically different fight formats.

At the time it was hard to find a local Krav Maga teacher. Some research on my part revealed that there was only one certified Krav Maga instructor in all of the Netherlands. Then a strange and serendipitous thing happened: a newly certified Krav Maga instructor rented the gym located at my University! I signed up immediately. I got my roommate to sign up too. For the first month, there were only three students. This made for a good pupil/teacher ratio.

Once I found an instructor and started taking Krav Maga classes, MMA started to lose its attraction. My martial Mind became fixated on self-defense scenarios. I would run imaginary situations over and over in my head. How would I deal with having a knife pulled on me? How about a club attack from behind? What about a bar fight? A street mugging where I was jumped by multiple attackers? How best to prevent or effectively finish a fight as soon as possible? Just as karate faded into MMA, MMA was fading in favor of Krav Maga.

I developed a real passion for this magnificent self-defense system. I disengaged from my fledging MMA path. Though initially torn, once it was done, it was a relief. I now had a lot of time back. I could redirect all my MMA time towards improving my quality of life. Things lightened up and improved immediately and dramatically. I have never regretted not pursing an MMA career.

Krav Maga is a way of dealing with deadly aggression in life or death situations. Krav Maga is two Hebrew words "contact combat." Krav Maga is a military self-defense system developed for the Israel Defense Forces (IDF) and used by the Israeli security forces, the Shin Bet and Mossad.

Krav Maga traces its roots back to Czechoslovakia in the mid-1930s. Hitler was the new leader of Germany and had many admirers and sympathizers in Czechoslovakia. In Bratislava, Hitler supporters were emboldened and would cruise the Jewish quarter of the city looking to physically assault or murder any Jew unlucky enough to cross paths with a roving band of drunken Nazi street thugs.

Imi Lichtenfeld lived in Bratislava. He was a Hungarian and happened to be a superb boxer and a bone-breaking wrestler. He devised the earliest form of Krav Maga. He taught it to Jewish residents to deal with being jumped or mugged, often by multiple Nazi attackers armed with clubs, knives, chains and guns. Imi emigrated to Israel in the 1940s and was asked to teach combat fighting to what was to become the IDF. Krav Maga expropriated simple and practical techniques from other fighting styles and created a philosophy that is simultaneously defensive and offensive.

Krav Maga was born in war: invented by commando Jewish partisans hunted by the Nazi SS. Commandos taught killing arts to members of the partisan underground. In addition to the actual physical drills associated with Krav Maga, there was also a sophisticated philosophy of usage. There are certain core principles that both define and differentiate Krav Maga from other martial arts. The founders of Krav Maga were intellectual warriors, men that fought and died perfecting the foundation upon which everything subsequent is constructed.

Krav Maga Principles
So that one may walk in peace

- **FLUIDITY;** keep evolving: Krav Maga does not resist change, it embraces change. Krav Maga is a reality-based self-defense method. Never static, always in motion, Krav Maga is in a state of continuing evolution. If we find a better and safer way to respond, we adopt it. Threats change. Long ago swords were common, today we have guns. Krav Maga seeks to provide the best possible solution.

- **EFFECTIVE,** efficient, sophisticated yet simple: Inflict maximum damage as rapidly as possible. Minimum time spent, minimum harm to self. End all fights as quickly as possible. Krav Maga techniques are designed for real life situations. Krav Maga is designed to train the individual to perform optimally under optimal stress.

- **KRAV MAGA** is for all levels: Everybody can and should learn Krav Maga. Regardless the individual's starting point, Krav Maga hones skills and spurs growth. No talent or special background needed. Krav Maga adjusts to your abilities.

- **BETTER YOURSELF:** Only compete with yourself. Krav Maga is not about ego. There is no competition. We need our training partners to help improve our skills. The group improves personal development. We do not compete with our training partners—we appreciate them. The enemy is not in our class.

- Aim for progression, not perfection
- In combat and in training—don't get hurt!
- Have a goal: continually refocus on your goal
- Intensity: finish the fight as soon as possible
- Pro-active: Avoid a fight if you can
- Always be aware of your surroundings
- Learn to switch between focus and awareness
- Trust your instructor and believe in yourself
- Do not comply with any sport or competition rules

I discovered that there was an entire library of Krav Maga techniques and tactics that I was completely unaware of—the more I learned the more I wanted to learn. Krav Maga placed a high value on intuitive response to stimuli, Krav Maga delved into the psychological aspects of self-defense. There is a definitive martial mindset, a mindset optimal for dealing with pressure. The optimal mindset is the absolute opposite of the frozen, confined mindset taught when adhering to a lone martial fighting style. I invented a specific mindset. Later I gave this mindset a name: the Krav Mindset.

Within a school or style, the classical mode of teaching is "when this attack occurs, counter with this counter strike or submission." The problem is in real combat things happen too quickly for the defender to mentally sort through the catalog of counter-attack possibilities. Krav Maga trains you to be intuitive and instinctual and respond with flow and fluidity to situations as they arise. Avoid the rigid and mechanical martial mindset—that all goes out the window when punched in the face or kicked in the groin. In a real-life scenario you need to cope with chaos, uncertainties and extreme stress. I decided to dedicate my life to spreading the word about this incredible self-defense system.

PRACTICAL FITNESS TRAINING

At the university, they had a gym in one of the buildings and as a student I could train there for a low price. It was a gym full of fitness machines. During my time in the army I got to know these resistance and cardio machines. At the university, part of the curriculum was "strength training," using the various progressive resistance machines. The type of strength produced by these machines was sadly lacking. All resistance machines are isolative, that is, they will work a single muscle at a time and never the entire body. Machines confine the user to little movements seldom used in real life. The body works best as a unit, coordinated and synchronized.

The classical bodybuilder approach strings together a series of isolation exercises, done set after set, using high reps and getting "a pump." This "muscle for muscles sake" approach always left me cold and wanting more. I did find one use for the resistance machines: I would perform a single high-rep set until I could not complete another safe repetition; then I would immediately move onto another machine and do the same thing. Then another and another, with no rest between sets. I might perform ten different exercises using ten different machine in a non-stop fashion.

At the end of the session my muscles would be blasted and my heart pounding through my chest. Now this was the type of workout I could relate to: a combination of muscular stress combined with intense cardio. When used in bodybuilding style, going for a pump, I did not like the effect the machines had on my body. Any "strength increases" registered on these machines were just poundage or rep increases applicable only on these machines. Everything was done sitting or lying down: I didn't care about pump strength created by these machines, I wanted the violent, explosive strength, the type Bruce Lee demonstrated with his famous "one-inch punch."

Machine training did not produce the athletically applicable strength that I needed in fighting and in life. I felt that the more machine training I did, the clumsier my movements became and the more my hand and foot speed slowed. Did handling more poundage or doing more reps in the lying leg curl or lat pulldown really improve my fighting performance? I got better at doing lying leg curls and lat pulldowns—but that didn't help my Krav Maga one iota.

By comparison I felt that the endless number of squats and lunges done in the military, all the while wearing a heavy backpack (increasing the intensity) had been far more effective at producing the type of integrated sustained strength I sought. During my commando training I had to do regular military fieldwork and this incredibly intense training had given me powerhouse legs; legs that had strength *and* stamina. I could kick like a mule and run all day long... what could be better?

As part of commando training, every single day we were made to squat, lunge, sprint and leap while going all out, 100%. And while wearing a heavy and awkward backpack. This type of strength-endurance work gave me applicable athletic power. My commando training was raw, simplistic, brutal, powerful and primitive. Machine training was (sometimes) fun but mostly boring and always ineffectual.

Machines are seductive. After my first disenchantment with machines, I swore them off. Several years later I was seduced again. I began training at a porch and upscale gym. The machines there were gorgeous: fancy and beautiful, comfortable to sit on or lie on. The gym had a nice-looking training room with lots of charm. So, yet again, I fell for the seductive charms of the glistening machines. After a month of zero progress I had a revelation: how can sitting down while training be even superficially beneficial?

I wanted the opposite, I wanted primitive and brutal training. I started training hard with hard men in hard gyms. I stopped frequenting the machine gyms. It was time for me to revisit Old School. Here is one workout routine that I did a lot of when in university. This routine was done when I first became immersed in Krav Maga. It combines sprinting with technique training. Bodyweight strength exercises alternated with speed-recovery drills to create contrast.

- Sprint 20 to 40 meters all out.
- Immediately begin jumping push-ups off the knuckles.
- Continue until just before form breaks down.
- Commence the active recovery phase with two minutes of fast-as-possible shadow boxing.
- Recover for one minute.
- Repeat the cycle 4-5 times in 30-minutes.

I would start this drill by sprinting 20 meters as fast as I could, from one wall to the other. No warm-ups! You don't get to warm-up when jumped by muggers. I would then sprint back to the starting line and immediately commence a bodyweight grind exercise.

You will find additional information about this section and the Krav Mindset at:

I did a lot of different knuckle push-ups. I really liked horizontal jumps. I went for distance and tried to jump 1.5 to 2 meters in distance, standing, with two feet together. I would turn 180-degrees while in the air, repeat until I could not make a one-meter distance. I would finish by leaping and shadow boxing, emphasizing hand and foot speed.

I have used variations of this sprint/grind/speed template for decades. With every round of shadow boxing, I would hide any visible fatigue as much I could—all part of increasing my mental strength. Fighting through fatigue teaches a fighter how to maintain proper posture.

Kettlebells were not available in those days. Kettlebell drills would have been easy to implement. Active recovery exercises completed the drill: I favored shadow boxing or rapidly repeating Dry-Drill Krav Maga techniques. Between each cycle I would rest until I felt I was ready to go again, usually about one minute. I repeated the drill. These workouts, done at lunchtime, lasted no longer that 30 minutes and were incredibly demanding.

I felt mentally revitalized and internally rewarded after these balls-out 30-minute sessions. Every time I was finished, I felt that I had extended myself and improved myself, physically and psychologically. I challenged and extended myself mentally. This mental satisfaction was something I had really missed while seduced at the "fitness gym." Being somewhat of a fitness fanatic, while everybody else was having their lunch or copying each other's homework, I was training.

Some guys with martial arts backgrounds noticed this dude training like crazy during lunch and being that they were also crazy, they wanted to join me for my lunch hour workouts. This was really fun. With training partners, we could expand the drills. The partner-drills were incredibly taxing.

We would do stuff like carry each other back and forth from one side of the room to the other. We sparred with one another during the active recovery speed phase. The principles of the workouts always stayed the same: intensive work interspersed with active recovery. The great thing was that there was never competition between us. We loved working out together. The goal was not to best or beat one another—the goal was to increase personal performances.

We all had different martial arts backgrounds and were different in size, build and fitness level. This made every training session rewarding and fun. Training together without the need to compete against each other was of great value. I carry this ideal with me to this day. As a side note, if you train for your own improvement, you don't need others to get you started and keep you going.

Working out in a group has great benefits. The atmosphere comes alive when people who are seeking the same thing come together: personal improvement. The group goal is to help individuals become a better version of themselves. Personal growth is the common goal. When training in a group, I discovered I could always go longer and effortlessly generate more intensity. I perform better with others working beside me. The idea is continual improvement. Krav Maga provides a superb overview as to how you get better every day.

This particular Krav Maga drill (sprint-grind-speed-recovery) is as result-producing today as it was way back when I first began doing it. Try cramming as many three-part drills as possible into 30-minutes. Any trainee that does this type of drill with the intensity and all-out effort it deserves will reap many tangible benefits: improved speed (sprinting,) improved power (push-ups or leaping squats) and improved cardio and agility (recovery sparring/shadow boxing.)

REALITY CHECK

After finishing my four years at the University, I now had a degree that would enable me to make a living pursuing a health and fitness-related career. During the same four-year period, I had also found my life's true passion, Krav Maga. Now what?

I was 24 years old, single, and I wanted to devote my life to Krav Maga, at least for the foreseeable future. Our experiences shape us. My unique background and my unique lifestyle choices led me to become instinctively and intuitively immersed in Krav Maga. I had fallen in love with a self-defense system. Because I could. I had lifted myself by my own bootstraps and found myself a totally free man. I could do what I want. I'd earned it.

I was young, capable, aggressive, if I wanted to do something crazy, like center my life around the pursuit of a martial art—then why not? I was beholden to no one. No wife, no children, no one I owed money to. I could get a real job teaching fitness. I could dedicate all my free time to my passion.

I really liked where I lived and had no desire to relocate. I lived in the university section of The Hague. After my bleak hometown and the harshness of the military, this environment was wonderful and productive. It was now familiar and had been my home for four years, the best four years of my life. I had friends and knew where to shop, how to get around and for the first time in my young life I was stress free, I was *happy*.

Because I had my degree I was qualified to teach in the public-school system. I thought that this was a viable career path. I admit that I was naïve. After living in the cloistered environment of college for four years, I had gotten out of touch with a lot of life's harsher realities. We didn't have crime or slums or poverty in the University neighborhood.

I became aware of a job opening in a secondary school, a high school, in a depressed suburb section of The Hague. I would be working with "troubled" students from arguably the worst section of town. Within this particular high school there was an ongoing series of gang wars; migrants battled the locals for supremacy within the school.

I interviewed. It would be a thirty-minute commute by car. No big deal. I had a car. Based on my age (older than most new teachers) my military background in special operations, and my martial skill set, I was hired right away. That should have been a tipoff. I got a quick starting date and reported for work not really knowing what to expect.

I am no stranger to downtrodden. I was downtrodden. My own childhood was bleak and deprived and it stayed that way until I joined the military. The army was no bed of roses either, populated by powerful alpha males that placed a premium on physicality. My four years at the University had detuned and diluted my street instincts. When a skill is not needed and not used it falls into disrepair: use it or lose it.

HIGH SCHOOL HELL

I had lost my instinctual street smarts and didn't even know it. On day one of the new job I was completely unprepared for the coarseness, rudeness, the disrespectful behavior displayed by students towards faculty and staff. This initial exposure to the widespread, commonplace use of vile gutter language was like a slap across the face.

I had come from the University, a world of civility and polite discourse; now I felt as if I been duped: hired as a teacher, seeking to share the wonders of fitness with eager students when in fact I was a prison guard at an institution full of dangerous inmates. This was a huge school with almost 2,000 students.

The students were hard and stone faced, 12 to 18 years old. Standing up to authority, i.e. the teachers and administrators, was considered a badge of honor and improved the student's status within the tribe.

The alpha male students set the tone of disrespect. Experience had shown that there would be no serious punishment for disrespect, even for the most egregious behavior. Past some sort of verbal reprimand, nothing would happen. The drop-out rate at the school was astronomical. The building was shabby and the whole place felt bleak, grey and depressing.

My first day impression was one of utter and complete chaos. Periods of relative quiet (during classes) were interrupted by periods of complete mayhem: vandalism and graffiti were popular pass times, fights occurred every day (including females) food and objects were routinely thrown, insults and foul language routine and accepted.

Often teachers had to physically restrain students, breaking students apart that were fist-fighting one another. Several teachers had been punched while breaking up fights. Fights were becoming more common and teachers getting punched or kicked breaking up fights was becoming more common.

The defense the "children" used was accepted by the PC school authorities. The defense was, "In the heat of battle, I did not see the teacher, it is their fault for leaping into the fray. Had they not jumped in, no injury would have occurred." Once that rationale was accepted, teachers became less inclined to intercede.

On my sixth day of my new job I became involved in my first violent incident. While breaking up a fight, one of the fighters, jacked up and enraged, did not like me pulling him off an undersized opponent. He was a man/boy bully mauling a child. He elbowed me hard in the gut when I grasped him from behind to pull him off. He then spun around, squared up and launched a powerful overhand right. I am quite sure he had used this punch to knock out many smaller weaker boys.

My first instinct was to set this bully on his back so hard it would knock him unconscious. I slid left and easily deflected his punch. Rather than deliver the vicious counter I so badly wanted to use in retaliation, I selected a simple choke slam (applied gently) that had him on the ground and on his back with my knee on his chest, all inside two seconds. In Krav Maga this is called an "educational block." I saw the pure fear in his eyes morph into anger: he knew because he was a "minor" I had done all the law would allow. "Get off me you child molester!" he hissed.

The frequency of incidents gradually escalated. When you get the reputation as the teacher that stands up to the bullies, you become a bully magnet, a benchmark. Confronting me, at least verbally, became a way to enhance street credibility. This sudden immersion into this strange new world of negativity triggered all kinds of repressed bully memories in me.

As a young boy I was small a favored target for bullies. The modern bullies I was confronting were the modern versions of my ancient tormentors. Many times, I had dreams in which I was small again, but possessing all the martial skills I do as an adult. In these dreams I would "set things right" and would envision old confrontations with new outcomes. Little Martijn would use his Krav Maga to devastate bullies from the past.

Mentally, while at school, I had to be on guard at all time. I could not let old demons influence current actions: my responses needed to be minimal and smothering—not devastating and deadly—as would be the case if I were jumped in the street by attackers with weapons. How easy it would be to "accidently" give some high school street punk, a bully disguised as a high school student, what he deserves: a swift, extremely hard, life-altering kick in the groin. "Allow me to introduce you, Mr. Bully, to a small dose of pain that you so freely and viciously administered to weaker, smaller boys over these many years..." I would be fired in a heartbeat.

But no, were I to unleash a full-scale counterattack, the "child" would end up hospitalized and I would end up institutionalized. Those that dared cross the line with me always got more than they bargained for. My response meter was set on its lowest setting. If you know your Krav Maga, you understand how easy it is to apply an excruciating counter attack, one that makes a strong man scream and beg—and in the next instant morph into a "soft-technique" without any harm or damage done, no marks left, no blood, no evidence of any kind of a physical encounter.

I would clamp on a bone lock and add a jolt of pain to amplify the message. I would release the hold before anyone could see what happened. The bone lock counters were reserved for the largest and meanest of the older boys, a clique that enjoyed extorting lunch money, stealing and preying on the youngest, smallest boys. The larger older bullies got my special time and attention.

REAL WORLD WORKSHOP

These periodic encounters with real world violence served as a report card for my ongoing Krav Maga evolution. Though it was not my intention, at a very formative and important time in my Krav Maga career (and the only time since) I was thrust into very real situations ending in spontaneous violence. There is the abstract world of martial theory and there is the devil's workshop of real world violence. The goal of every martial arts is to allow adherents to prevail in a real-world fight, a spontaneous, violent, life-threatening situation.

Krav Maga was never a sport. Krav Maga is a combat fighting system designed to counter attacks from individuals or groups of attackers. By now, at age 24, I was a full-fledged Krav Maga instructor. My Krav Maga obsession took up all my free time. I either taught or studied Krav Maga. I felt I had broken through to another level in my own martial arts competency. The essence of the teachings became second nature; I discovered there was no substitute for practice and reps and mental imaging. Krav Maga's intended purpose is dealing with reality: how do we deal with truly violent situations?

Periodically, I was encountering violent incidents of varying intensities. The Krav Maga I had learned had now been taken deep into my marrow. It was serving me well in those totally spontaneous, instantaneous real-life violent situations. Krav Maga was delivering on its promise—and why not?

MY 15 MINUTES OF FAME

A STRANGE DETOUR ON MY LIFE'S JOURNEY

In 2005 I started my first website. I began posting articles on why I thought that everybody should learn Krav Maga. The internet offered an easy platform and a way in which to reach the widest possible audience for next to no cost. I dutifully made a few YouTube Krav Maga demo videos and posted them.

Past that, I didn't think too much about them. I had low expectations. I was in my second year of teaching at high school when one evening in 2007 I got a call from a man that had been surfing the internet and came across my Krav Maga website. After some initial conversation, he related that he was a producer for a new Dutch reality TV show. Would I be interested in becoming a cast member on a reality TV show?

The show would be shooting a pilot season, seven episodes done in Kenya. Filming would take seven weeks. The theme of the show would be skilled adults, of whom I would be one, working with "troubled teens" in a purposefully primitive environment.

Could the combination of Nature, depravation, expert adult counseling, discipline and love turn the teens around in seven weeks? I was already dealing with "troubled teens" on a daily basis and I was extremely skeptical that something miraculous could happen in 49 days.

Seven teenagers would be removed from their current toxic home environments and placed in a camp in Kenya, in a naturalistic setting. This would be like a military boot camp combined with therapy session. Could these youngsters be cured and corrected? Could exposure to nature and primal living and stern advice allow them to dissipate their anger and direct their frustration and rage into a more constructive life? Could we save teenagers headed towards a life of crime, jail, gangs or death? Could their lives be turned around? That was the premise as it was presented to me.

The crapshoot was—would it work out? Just because you bring a bunch of kids and counselors and a film crew to Kenya doesn't guarantee that at the end of seven weeks you are going to have a bunch of radically changed boys and girls. You could spend all that time, effort and money by the barrelful—and at the end the kids could still be the same jerks and bullies they were to begin with.

The kids selected were not picked because they got good grades and behaved themselves. They got picked because they were flamboyant, prone to act out (makes for good TV) and one step away from incarceration. It was one hell of a gamble. Can you imagine how much money it took to transport and house twenty people, all on payroll, to Kenya for seven weeks?

There were other questions: would there be enough weekly action to make for interesting viewing during the seven-week process? Just because the producers wanted the series to be perfect—seven teens start off horrid, disgusting, disrespectful and stupid beyond belief and are transformed into model children—and all in seven short weeks. Standing back and looking at this dispassionately, I would think maybe one or two out of these seven delinquent kids could be turned around.

I was asked if I would be interested in interviewing to become an on-camera cast member. It would require an eight-week time commitment. I was being interviewed to become the leading camp instructor that lived 24-7 with the troubled teens. I interviewed and obviously they liked my unique background, i.e. I was former troubled kid, plus I had been a commando, a self-defense instructor and I was a school teacher teaching troubled teens. I had youth and fitness. I was selected.

I became a cast member on the Dutch reality TV show Van Etter tot Engel Goes Kenya. Surprisingly, I did not have too hard a time obtaining a leave of absence from the high school. Being selected made me distinctive and helped my peer status in the teacher profession immensely. How many people get asked to appear in a seven-week reality TV show set in Kenya? I got the impression that they were rather proud that one of their own was selected.

I took a leave of absence and not knowing what to expect, I traveled to Kenya and was transported to our permanent camp site, fifty miles outside of Nairobi. It was a true jungle encampment. The campsite had been hacked out of the jungle by Masai tribesmen. They warned us to be alert; periodically elephants would stampede through our campsite.

One day I saw a cheetah bring down a gazelle while standing outside my tent. Another morning I woke up, finding a big pile of shit, just in front of my tent. It seemed that a hippo left it there during the night. I loved primal primitive nature. I loved the landscape and I loved the wildlife. This was the real deal.

The camp counselors and the troubled teens lived in tents and ate local food that they had to prepare themselves. The film crew and TV producer types (a dozen) lived in different tents and ate catered meals fifty yards away. The kids were hardcore. Naturally, unless there is drama, unless the troubled teens acted out and created chaos then there is not much of a show. No one tunes into a reality TV show to see normal kids act normal.

That would be a very boring show. No, the TV viewing audience wants to see kids punching adults, kids breaking car windows with rocks, kids running away, kids stealing, kids hot wiring, stealing and wrecking cars and being hateful while using profane language. Then with time, nature and our expert counseling, these spiteful, hateful, mean kids will be transformed into law-abiding citizens, cured of all bad habits and evil ways.

Seven kids, five counselors and seven straight weeks with no breaks... We got the kids detoxed, physiologically and psychologically. It worked. (of course!) Taken out of their toxic groove and being deposited in the jungle for a protracted period will change anyone.

It certainly changed me. I took to it. The kids did not. Many city and suburban kids do not like hardcore Nature and had a hard time being in nature. While outdoorsmen (like me) see beauty in wildlife and sunsets, these city kids see bugs and snakes and deadly beasts and are perpetually frightened and freaked out.

There was a deadening sameness, a boredom and repetitiveness that caused a lot of upset and consternation initially. Most eventually stopped fighting and got with the program. Naturally, the most interesting episodes involved the teens that held out the longest and acted out the most.

After weeks and weeks of intense isolation, the poison and toxicity that fueled the kids anger and frustration finally exhausted itself. Only then could we talk sense to them and have them hear it. We (the adult cast members) preached the same message of moderation and saneness from day one, but for most it took weeks and weeks before they heard the logic in the message. Which was, basically, be smart and act in your own best self-interest. Don't hurt others. Use your street smarts in society. Channel and focus. Naturally it made for riveting TV.

The seven episodes aired shortly after we returned. Within six months my students and faculty members were seeing me on weekly episodes. It was surreal seeing myself. I was the camp counselor that would jump in when things got physical, violent or things started getting thrown. I was told I was selected because of my self-defense skills and that the TV people fully expected some of the kids would get physical and would need to be restrained from hurting others or themselves. As expected, there were numerous instances where I had to interpose myself between two teens or a teen and an adult.

Many of the "children" were certified bullies that frequently resorted to violence to get their way or impose their will on the weaker and smaller back in their world. Now, here in the jungle, the human predators naturally attempted to play their games on the other teens. Back in their world, there were no martial arts experts continually in their presence, ready to shut down any and all aggression. Naturally the TV audience loved it when a kid got worked up to such a degree that he had to be subdued and restrained—by me. My role was clear.

The producers and the viewing audience fell in love with my Krav Maga. I could ratchet down my responses to such a degree that there was never any harm done to any teen. I would simply step in front of them and wait for them to make an aggressive offensive move towards me. Be it a punch or a kick, I would smother the blow and convert it into a rip, a sweep or a bone-lock. Which always ended it. I don't care who you are, if you are caught in a restraining hold by a Krav Maga expert you will cooperate.

I would confront the teen that was threatening violence or being violent. I would intercept the blow and usually use a leg sweep to take them to the ground. However, when I want to take an opponent down in a real fight with a violent criminal, I would take the opponent down hard, amplified with all my bodyweight or a knee or a fist. When I swept a teen, I would actually hang onto them, preventing them from impacting the ground hard. I would then follow them down, usually establishing the neutral, knee-on-chest dominant position while I grasped each wrist. Now, face to face, they would see I had them totally checkmated. They invariably gave up when they realized I was toying with them.

I cannot tell you how many parents have come up to me after the shows had aired to express to me that they wished they'd had my martial skills when dealing with their own violence-prone children. Krav Maga allows me to modulate my response in direct proportion to the degree of the threat. I have a set of skills for neutralizing small children. I have another skill set for older, larger, stronger teens. I have a totally different intensity level when responding to a knife attack or an attempted car-jacking by an adult criminal.

We did our seven weeks in Kenya and filmed seven episodes. I loved my time in the jungle and being an animal-lover, I was in big beast paradise. I was surprised how quickly the episodes began appearing. A lot of people watched this show and it got good reviews. I thought I came across stern and humorless. Regardless, everyone in my orbit seemed to watch.

I made a nice amount of money, I was paid well for my time away from home. Back home it felt weird to me to be recognized by strangers and weirder yet to be asked for an autograph. I was back to my regular life at the high school, breaking up fights and confiscating marijuana. I didn't feel special or star-like, except for the next year I could not go anywhere or do anything where someone didn't recognize me. So strange. Then things got even stranger.

A year after the seven episodes of Van Etter tot Engel aired, I was approached by another reality TV show, a much bigger show funded by the Dutch Public Broadcasting System. Essentially, I would reprise my role as referee/enforcer in a different format. The show was called Family Matters.

At its peak, we had one million viewers a week, huge numbers for Dutch TV. This time six emotionally-troubled teens and their parents were quarantined with six counselors for three weeks. The show had plenty of everything that makes for exciting TV. The characters selected were a volatile mix, purposefully selected to grate on one another until someone exploded. Which coincidentally happened every episode. Personally, I thought that the parents were far more obnoxious and screwed up than the kids.

We stayed in the Pyrenees Mountain region, in the geographic saddle between Spain and France. It was a beautiful location, rustic and picturesque—but it was no Africa. I missed the majestic beauty of jungle and beast. The participants were continual trouble and in episode after episode I end up having to lay hands on someone. A favored tactic was to throw rocks through windows and break up property.

I had one situation that was very serious that almost got a full-on adult response. One troublemaker decided to take his acting out to the next level. I'd already had several hands-on confrontations with this punk. He knew he did not stand a chance fighting me and I had embarrassed him several times and caused him to lose face. He knew how easily I countered any blow he launched my way. Those same blows had hurt a lot of smaller, weaker children back in his habitat. Now here he was, frustrated and hell-bent on revenge.

This time he decided he use a weapon. He attacked me with a brick. He intended to smash my face with the brick. I stop-blocked his brick hand, dislodging the brick, sending it flying. I ripped him to the ground in a flash. I almost gave him a full-on throat shot, as I would have had he been a weapon-wielding adult. I thankfully checked my instantaneous instinct and ground his face into the ground, perhaps a bit too enthusiastically.

While the African show was successful, the second reality show, Family Matters, was a runaway smash hit. Now I was more recognized than ever.

After the ratings success of Family Matters, plans were immediately hatched for the next season. It would be filmed around the same time that my wife and I were expecting our second child. I just needed to be there for my son's birth, so I had to decline. My son Jonas was born in 2011.

This second season turned out to be another success story so they planned a third season. This time the scenario would shift gears and we would counsel four women with eating disorders.

Filmed in Spain, the cast and crew were reunited. Our expectations were sky high. The feeling was we were on the verge of creating a long-running reality TV series. I had visions of quitting teaching and getting a new car within a year.

Filming began. The new scenario was offbeat: teenage girls with eating disorders, accompanied by their parents. This was a totally different vibe. No alpha male thugs to act out. Four females were fully capable of throwing tantrums, but female ranting and raging was of a different type and flavor.

It was difficult for me; my prime role had been as the alpha male enforcer, a man whose main function was to subdue alpha teens when they smashed the plate glass window with a rock and started running down the highway.

The question again was, could we, the staff, get these girls healed and straightened out in the time allotted? The mostly odious parents made a bad situation worse. They continually interfered, offering unsolicited, awful advice on a habitual basis.

The TV people wanted to create tension and angst that would boil over and blow up. Then, the expert staff would step in, fix and heal everyone in time for a tidy and timely ending to our eight-week, eight-episode series. The TV people wanted explosive results that would make for riveting TV and they got that—but not the type and kind anyone expected.

After the filming, a day before the press viewing, the project was cancelled to air. A sexual abuse charge was leveled against the male star of our series. He was accused of attacking one of the participants. All hell broke loose.

It ended what could have potentially be the start of a promising career as a reality TV star.

Worse still, it became a huge tabloid and TV scandal. The salacious nature of the crime and the high profile of the show ensured it was all over the newspapers and TV. It was a nightmare. Worst of all, I was tarred by association.

There was a suddenness about it that left me confused and angry. I went from minor celebrity with a 'good guy' aura to somehow tainted and part of a national sex scandal. Imagine having TV crews and reporters following you around, asking things like, "Why didn't you stop the abuse?" Can you imagine? I am a regular person. Now suddenly I am hounded by reporters having microphones shoved in my face.

I had never even met a reporter, now I am being asked, "Can you comment on why you did not see this coming? Did you know about this? Why didn't you do something to prevent this? You and the star were best friends—were you not?" I wanted to launch and starting ranting. Not a smart idea. So, I would say, "No comment."

I had had visions of making enough off the reoccurring reality TV series to stop teaching and devote myself to Krav Maga. I could see myself making that kind of money in the not-too-distant future. I cannot convey how popular this series was. If you go to YouTube, you can find clips, though it is in Dutch. All that evaporated and went up in smoke.

Apparently, I'd had my fifteen minutes of fame and was now cast out. Those were three wild and exciting years.

Like Sisyphus, the boulder that was my media career rolled back down to the bottom of the hill. I had to begin from zero. I was forced to go back to grinding it out as a high school teacher. I was living a bad dream. I was back in an old groove, a crushing, deadening groove, I was a fallen star sucked back into the drudgery of his old reality.

SECONDARY SCHOOL PURGATORY AND TAKING THE PLUNGE

It would be nice to say that, after two years teaching secondary school, I witnessed and was part of a dramatic solution that cured all the misery, poverty and crime that plagued the high school I taught at. Nothing changed during my years teaching within this impoverished school district. Our low graduation rate was low when I arrived and stayed low, parents were mostly absentee, petty crime, vandalism and drugs (both hard and soft) were as plentiful and prolific when I left as when I showed up.

True, we had some small victories during my two-year tenure. I engineered a national grant that resulted in a lot of help and financial aid for the school and for its least fortunate students. I had to navigate a mountain of paperwork and by doing so and be being steadfast I was able to obtain a block grant that gave real people in real need real money. In the end, the causes for the crime and poverty were as strong (if not stronger) when I left as they were when I showed up.

Simultaneous to teaching at school on a full-time basis, I was teaching Krav Maga almost every night. I got a job as instructor at the gym I used to train at in The Hague. After teaching for a year, I started a gym on my own. In order to avoid any conflict of interest, I opened my Krav Maga studio in my home town of Alphen ad Rijn, 60-minutes from the gym where I taught Krav Maga. I could not be accused of picking off students, or in any way competing with the people I was working for.

I had taken on so much and was committed in so many ways that I felt nothing was as good as it should be. During this time, still a teacher, I plotted my next move. I had no intention of making a career out of teaching at secondary school. Ultimately, optimally, I wanted to spread the word of Krav Maga and empower people. I wanted to be a fulltime Krav Maga professional. To get to that point would take careful planning. I needed to be in business for myself. I would morph from secondary school teacher into full-time Krav Maga instructor. I would own my own gym. That might take a while. In the meantime, I would need to keep a foot in each world. I was young and I could take the pace.

FORMULATING PHILOSOPHIES

First and foremost, I wanted a single-purpose martial arts facility, a facility dedicated totally and completely to Krav Maga. This would be completely new in The Netherlands. I did not have any examples to follow. There were some kickboxing gyms in Holland, but they were using the faces of some famous world champions. Nobody knew anything about Krav Maga at that time and that was a huge downside.

I saw opportunity: commercial martial arts studios are in every major town over 50,000 from California to Moscow. I felt that Krav Maga, with its utilitarian purpose, could and would get traction with the wider populace. It just needed time and exposure. I remember Bruce Lee once said he wanted to build as many Kung-Fu schools as there were McDonalds. His point being that everyone everywhere is entitled to be schooled in self-defense. I wanted what Bruce wanted, but I wanted more.

I wanted to create a trainings center that would offer a wide array of interrelated disciplines: the foundational discipline would be Krav Maga—but augmented by my new strength training method. I wanted to further develop this unique brand of strength training. I wanted my strength training protocols to amplify the Krav Maga skill set.

Nowadays a lot of gyms offer both fitness and self-defense lessons. I was the first in my area to meld fitness training with Krav Maga. I had a vision for my training center, improvement of both physical *and* mental, physiological and psychological. My facility would have a philosophy and purpose.

I wanted to maintain my lifestyle, one that was hardly lavish or opulent. I lived in a messy little apartment in a clean and exciting section of The Hague. The goal was to achieve critical mass in my business; make enough money off teaching Krav Maga and strength training that I would be able to quit teaching.

My Krav Maga student retention was incredible. The best advertisement for your business are transformed and empowered students. They become unpaid advertising for your effectiveness. Word of mouth by enthused students bought me 70% of my new students. Slowly, methodically I added more and more new members.

It was a tall order with a lot of potential pitfalls. I needed to build a Krav Maga student base with enough critical mass to pay the bills. It was a big leap from being a public servant with a regular paycheck to the high-wire act of owning a commercial business. I sought to create a self-sustaining business, one based on a self-defense system that no one knew about.

My remarkable retention rate was due to the art itself. Once people were introduced to Krav Maga, once they got it, they fell in love with it and stayed with it. Krav Maga is sensible in that it is rooted in science and logic and hard-won empirical battle experience, first with resistance fighters after WWII and later with the IDF as their combat fighting art.

Over time I refined my business plan. I needed to generate enough gross income teaching Krav Maga that I could afford to rent a studio, invest in training materials and local promotion while creating a cadre of solid students: ones that were dedicated and behaved correctly, both in and outside my class. I wanted my own studio(s) and did not want to practice my art under someone else's roof, and certainly not using someone else's philosophy.

I had trained in enough gyms, dojos, fight clubs and studios to know what I wanted. I needed my own place I could use every night. I needed instructors to teach alongside with me, to help me offer more lessons. The totality of it shaped me. I had a lot at stake. Financially, if the businesses failed I would be in dire straits. One of the advantages of being in perpetual motion is you don't have a lot of time to dwell on the negative. At night, I would pass out exhausted and fall into a satisfied, deep, dreamless sleep.

It was during the same time that my wife and I were expecting our first child. I met Suzanne in Kenya. She was the producer of the reality TV show. She was intelligent, humorous, way smarter than me and a successful professional. I don't know what she saw in me. In the beginning, neither did she. We came from such different worlds and had such differing backgrounds. Yet there was undeniable chemistry. I married her in 2008. Suzanne is a caring woman with a mind of her own. My teaching four nights a week for years on end wasn't ideal for our relationship, but she let me do my thing. She never tried to stop me from chasing my dream. When she was at home, I was working late. She knew a bit about my background, accepted my passion and kept supporting me. Lucy was born in 2009.

HOGESCHOOL

In 2006 I applied for a new and exciting job. I interviewed and was offered a fulltime position teaching "sports science" at Hogeschool Inholland. This school was in a nice area and I would be teaching substantial subjects like physiology, didactics, conflict resolution and conflict adhesion. Real topics taught to students that cared. These were College level students. No one was in my class that was not there voluntarily. I sailed through the interview process and was hired.

The university teaching environment was perfect: I was in a low stress situation instructing students that were respectful and engaging. It was a revelation to enjoy coming to work. Instead of intellectually stunted, I was now intellectually stimulated.

I purchased my first house with Suzanne. It was located just 15 minutes from my new job at the University in Haarlem. My new home was a full fifty minutes' drive from my longtime flat in The Hague.

After I got moved into the new home, I took my Krav Maga business to the next level. To make a long story short, after two years of renting a facility for two nights a week, my client base had reached critical mass. I now was making enough money to be able to rent a really nice facility 24-7-365 and decorate to my tastes.

This was a big deal for me and a major turning point: Krav Maga was getting traction. Now, in addition to working a fulltime teaching job, I taught five days a week at one of two studios.

From the time I opened my eyes at 6 am until I went to bed eighteen hours later, I would spin from one important task to another. For the next four years I worked two jobs in three different locations six days a week. I segregated my life into segments and attacked each new task as it arose.

First and foremost, I needed to perform up to (and past) expectations on my new job at the university. The teaching job was the foundation of everything good going forward, as it represented a considerable increase in my paycheck and a considerable reduction in my stress levels. I really liked the environment and I really liked the faculty and students. I found it easy to give 110% while teaching at the Hogeschool.

I also needed to adjust my relationship with the students. I taught a compulsory fitness class and my natural tendency was for me to be a tad harsh. I needed to chill a bit. Coming from a tough high school full of delinquents, I had developed a new and more civil and appropriate persona. That prison guard persona was not appropriate for my new school.

As a group these students were intelligent, well spoken, decent, earnest types. They had a different kind of shortcoming. Where my previous students lacked respect for authority, these students lacked discipline. Whereas the high school students were arrogant and unrepentant, the college students were smart enough to adapt quickly to my rules.

The nonchalant attitude exhibited by the Hogeschool students initially irritated the hell out of me. I expressed it to them. Behind my back they called me, "Sargent Fury." I was the one that needed an attitude adjustment. These students were future health club owners and lifestyle professionals. I needed to realize that this wasn't Commando tryouts for an elite unit.

Teaching at the university was a pure joy. Imagine going from breaking up fist fights to spirited classroom discussions with bright people, eager students hungry for knowledge. This was the type of teaching environment I wanted to work in. Instead of dreading going to work, I looked forward to my new teaching position.

While outside of the school day I never had enough time, during the school day, I had long open periods of free time. Teachers were encouraged to use these gaps between classes to improve their academic skillset.

I took full advantage of these free period to research all the strength training academic studies I could find. I familiarized myself with all the latest cutting-edge strength training procedures and protocols. I now had time to mull over what I had read and hone own my philosophy of strength. I did this between classes.

I would then implement my newly formed abstract strength strategies, turning abstraction into the reality, in my training sessions. Specifically, I was intrigued with various academic studies that related to improving the five bio-motor skills: strength, speed, endurance, agility and flexibility.

As a teacher, as a fulltime fitness professional, as a Krav Maga instructor, as someone interested in improving my own performance and my own physique, it was only natural that I immerse myself in academic studies as it related to improving bio-motor capacities.

When developing and refining my Trojan Workout, I was particularly drawn to the premier bio-motor attribute, strength. Strength is the preeminent bio-motor attribute because strength is needed in the other bio-motor skills. There is no speed without strength. There is no sustained strength or strength endurance without strength. There are different types and kinds of strength.

At one strength extreme is the grinding isometric type of strength used when clinching or grappling, grind strength is used to muscle and overwhelm an opponent; at the other strength extreme is explosive strength best exemplified by punches and kicks that detonate on impact, shattering bones and knocking attackers' unconscious; explosive strength that manifests with body-shocking striking power.

Strength originates in the brain. The brain impulse shoots through the nervous system into the muscles. I remember a quote from Dan John; "The brain doesn't know anything about muscles." In some way it made sense to me that the brain is the origination point for both mental and physical strength. Strength is focus and intensity. You can't fake strength.

REAL LIFE EXPERIENCE

It was shortly after I had taken my new teaching position that during school break I went on holiday to Ibiza. I was out with a friend heading back to the hotel when four young men approached us. My warning senses went off immediately.

The leader of this little pack stepped forward and grabbed me by the arm while lifting his other arm as if to strike me. He told me loudly and profanely to hand over our wallets. It was an armed robbery and the way this group spread out left no doubt that this gang was skilled at sticking up tourists.

Instinctively and without any thought I blocked his arm punch and gave him a solid counter strike, a straight right hard to his face. In my Krav Maga classes I warned my students several times that in most cases, you won't see if an attacker has a knife. It's a sad thing but most survivors only realize after an incident that the attacker was using a knife when they see the holes in their body or suddenly feel something wet and sticky under their shirt. *If* they survive.

The moment I blocked the leader's arm and simultaneously countered with a punch in his face, I saw a huge knife dropping from out of his hand. Without my instantaneous block/hit I would have been slashed or stabbed.

The instant I saw the knife, it was on. Had they confined their robbery attempt to words or even rough stuff, I likely would have attempted to talk them out of it or scare them off. His first mistake was attacking me when he was within arms-length. His second mistake was his overconfidence.

Because he was so close to me I hit him flush on the nose, hard and suddenly. I used a counterstrike combination that I'd practiced a thousand times. It was a block/hit where simultaneous to the block I smashed the unprotected nose (and groin) mashing it flat, then hit him on the back of his head with the inside of my forearm.

He collapsed like he'd been shot. As was expected, the second-string leader of this little crime gang stepped up just in time for the crushing side-kick that sent him backwards and onto the beach sand. Also predictable was that now, since I'd coldcocked the overconfident leader and busted the ribs of the assistant boss, the other two took off. Two blows, two men needing hospitalization and all inside one minute.

Again, I really would have preferred to have avoided the whole incident, however it was gratifying that in real life situations Krav Maga works and works as promised. Again, it changed my life!

TRANSITIONING

For the four years I taught at the university, I was in perpetual motion. The totality of the activities and the degree of continual concentrated effort morphed me as a man and as an athlete; it morphed me mentally and it morphed me physically. I was continually subjected to what I would call 'performance pressure,' as opposed to the negative chronic stress.

Everything I was involved with I was enthused about and upbeat about. My performance pressures needed to be managed and focused and converted into across-the-board improved performance. I needed to get better at a lot of things simultaneously.

The unrelenting totality of the effort was draining and exhausting—and exhilarating. This was a critical period during which I formulated all the defining characteristics for the Trojan Workout. I developed my business and I developed my Krav Maga teaching style. Not all good athletes make good coaches. I was a good teacher. As a teacher during the day at college, or as a self-defense teacher, I evolved and improved my communicative skills. I got a lot of practice.

I found I needed to compartmentalize Krav Maga and Trojan Workout. I needed to divide Krav Maga in two halves: the business side and my own personal development as a student. I also had to find a way to keep doing strength training, even with a total lack of time. Without strength training my body would be more susceptible to impact injuries and chronic stress.

They say necessity is the mother of invention and out of necessity I created the concept of "habitual short workouts." This time compactness became a foundational principle for my newly minted Trojan Workout.

I needed a compressed strength training program that would keep my muscles strong, my neurological system performing optimally and all the while maintaining my natural durability, my ability to take a punch. I sought to keep my hormonal levels optimal; I sought to reduce my cortisol and elevate my growth hormone levels and testosterone levels.

My routine required that (for three straight years) I work seven days a week. Even writing it now makes me tired. Back then, it was one day at a time, one step forward, followed by another and another. From the time, I awoke until when I went to bed 18 hours later, I rotated from one important task to the next, from one scheduled time block to the next. It was an intensely challenging time. I needed to do it all and I needed to do it all right. No half work, as my mother used to say.

Not all my breakthroughs were physical, some were psychological. In about this time I formalized a way to consciously shift between two types of definable consciousness: focus and awareness. I taught students to recognize and differentiate between focus and awareness. I had a method for shifting between the two psychological perspectives.

Awareness is the overview, the soft eye that sees everything with a wide panoramic perspective. While awareness is wide and macro, focus is narrow and micro. Focus is contained in a narrow field of vision. Focus is the intense concentration needed to fend off an attack. Both focus and awareness are needed. My idea was to formalize a way to toggle back and forth between the two on an as-needed and when-appropriate basis.

During a violent confrontation, Krav Maga students are taught to not stay locked into the micro, narrow vision focus mode. This happens automatically when fending off an attack from someone right in front of you. This "locked in focus" mode makes you vulnerable to attack from a second attacker. The optimal approach is to rapidly shift from hard focus to soft-eye awareness, an ability which is a learned skill.

It was during this time that I formalized the precepts and principles that define the Trojan Workout. It took a lot of thought, a lot of experimentation and playing with the component parts. When I would get overwhelmed or confused by too many legitimate choices, I kept referring myself back to my original principles: what was the prime goal of the Trojan Workout? Stand strong! Build confidence, build strength in your body!

I made the Trojan Workout approachable and suitable for every individual. One aspect of Krav Maga that really appealed to me was that it was doable by all individuals at all levels. I wanted to replicate that in the Trojan Workout. Everybody can become stronger using Trojan Workout principles; everyone can learn self-defense using Krav Maga. In Krav Maga, many mental benefits are derived simply by showing up and putting in the work. I made sure to replicate this trait in the Trojan workout.

I had zero interest in bodybuilding strategies that created muscle without any real purpose other than vanity. I sought something totally different, something that I could not find. Necessity is the mother of intention and my necessity was to create a complimentary and comprehensive system of strength that provides usable, functional, athletically applicable physical strength AND also increase and improves mental strength.

I sought more than one type of strength. As a Krav Maga instructor, I wanted the manhandling abilities that come when a person develops grind strength. I also wanted the speed and knockout power that defines explosive strength. Thirdly I wanted the ability to exert power over protracted periods. Three types of strength. Every strength system I examined would champion one or perhaps two of the three definable strength types. I wanted all three to be addressed in the Trojan Workout.

Eventually it occurred to me that I needed to create a new strength system. Rather than continue on this never-ending chase to find a comprehensive strength system, one nuanced enough to incorporate all three strength types, the obvious solution was for me to create what I had in mind.

I needed to pay proper attention to all the varieties and types of strength. Once I began to teach the earliest versions of the Trojan workout, I monitored how it made my students feel. By doing this I could modulate the training intensities. The idea is to challenge but not break or injure the student. Make them stronger without hurting them. That which does not kill me makes me stronger.

I joined my newfound across-the-board-strength system to my Krav Maga. I envisioned the Trojan Workout creating dramatic breakthroughs in performance and radical improvements in physique and performance, regardless the drill selected. The Trojan Workout would increase lean muscle mass and reduce body fat. A stronger, leaner, fitter fighter is a far better fighter.

KETTLEBELL THUNDERBOLT

During my second year of teaching at university, I traveled to Hungary for a Krav Maga Law Enforcement course. The featured speaker was touting the explosive strength benefits of a new training tool: the kettlebell. The crudeness of the kettlebell instantly appealed to me: this ugly beast of a tool was the exact opposite of an expensive, isolative exercise machine found in the bodybuilding gyms.

The kettlebell master's presentation was excellent: he explained that by handling moderate poundage in an explosive fashion, usable athletic strength, functional strength, could and would be built. You could also use the kettlebell to create grind and isotonic intensities and finally the kettlebell could be used for protracted periods to create extended strength. With a few different weight kettlebells, all three strength types could be maximally taxed. My mind was on fire with the possibilities.

The demonstrator then got out the biggest kettlebell I'd ever seen in my life (a 104-pound "beast" kettlebell) and proceeded to perform a series of slo-mo grind movements. My head spun in circles thinking of how I could incorporate this new crude tool into my own emerging strength philosophy.

I became completely fascinated by the kettlebell. I had found the tool I needed to implement my formative strength training ideas and protocols. I had to make time for kettlebell training. So, I made time and it seemed like with every kettlebell session my knowledge doubled, my performance improved, and my body hardened. My very first kettlebell was a tiny 16-kilo toy.

I knew nothing at the time and learned all my kettlebell basics using this small kettlebell. In some ways, this was a good thing. I developed excellent techniques that I ingrained and retained, techniques I use and teach to this day. The bell allowed me to try some juggling, tossing and catching the bell, getting it airborne. Juggling is a useful and productive protocol that I would never have learned had I not been "stuck" with the 16 for all that time.

After a few months I figured out that the 16-k bell was too light to generate the strength results I sought. I moved to successively larger kettlebells and with each kettlebell poundage increase came outstanding gains in muscle, power and strength. Now I could replicate the grind approach, I could replicate the explosive strength tactics I had worked out in my head and on paper. If I wanted to develop the endurance of a long-distance runner, I could do so using a light bell for extended periods. One tool could deliver on a multitude of levels.

With the time I had on my hands between classes, I learned new things and would implement these new angles and approaches into my own training. I was my own laboratory. I solidified my core training philosophies during my tenure at university.

To improve martial skills the student needs to improve cardio, agility and mobility. My newly conceived Trojan Workout protocols now provided strength and speed. There is no speed without strength. When Krav Maga is practiced diligently and when Trojan workout and strength training are practiced diligently, both body and Mind improve. As we forge the body, we forge the mind.

THE RIGHT TOOL AT THE RIGHT TIME FOR THE RIGHT MAN: SLOW POWER IS NO POWER

I suppose you could say that "I got" kettlebells, and the philosophy behind kettlebells right away. I was lucky enough to see a kettlebell demonstration by a man that knew what he was doing. The explosive snap was apparent in the way in which they were demonstrated: this wasn't slow, ponderous lifting, this was crisp and explosive. Perfect techniques were stressed and demonstrated. I had never seen any strength exercise, ever, that resembled the kettlebell swing: the pop created by the hip snap was awesome. I loved the balletic Turkish get-up. Kettlebell pressing had a highly specific technique. The pistol squat was a revelation.

I felt kettlebells were the perfect tool for creating an effective strength system designed specifically for a practicing martial artist. My own research and my own fighting experience had led me to seek two specific strength types: grind (or isometric) strength and explosive strength. In my real world fighting experience, two types of strength were continually needed. The first is what I would describe as tight grappling; pulling, tugging or struggling with the opposing strength and the bodyweight of an opponent. Grip strength and grind power are needed. You assert your will, you overpower an opponent. You also need a body that can take a hit. The body can be built to absorb hits. We seek to build a body that can endure collisions.

The second type of strength sought is explosive strength. It is one thing to overpower an opponent in a clinch; it is quite another thing to be able to deliver a lightning fast blow that packs a wallop. That last part, packs a wallop, is critical. Lightning fast punches and kicks are wonderful but if they underpowered they will have no more effect than a slap. I was fast and skinny and my punches, no matter how hard I threw them, were light blows for big men. Back when I weighed 70 kilos my blows aggravated big men; nowadays at 85 kilos my blows knock big men unconscious.

Slow power is no power. A man can have a 500-pound bench press yet if his punch is slow, it is a push, not a punch. Optimally the fighter seeks to combine strength and speed to create true power. We seek the type of explosive power Mike Tyson has in his right uppercut. A punch that sent men careening over backwards. How best to acquire explosive power? Train explosively! Krav Maga aims for the body's most vulnerable points, so that any attack is effective. The more explosive strength you possess, the greater the fist or foot impact. Strong stacks up well, even against much bigger opponents. A strong body performs better than a weak body when stressed. And a strong body looks better.

The kettlebell, as a tool and a protocol, would become a big part of my life from this point forward. My own bio-motor research kept leading me towards strength. For most of my life I had to contend with being undersized and underpowered. I found I could neutralize larger stronger opponents by being faster, more agile and possessing better cardio. I also had a high pain tolerance. In those years teaching at the university I gained 10 kilos of bodyweight, all of it solid muscle.

The difference in my power and strength after training for a while with kettlebells was astounding. To be the best possible Kravist, in addition to being skillful within my art, I vowed to work on the bio-motor attributes that would contribute to my being a better conditioned, stronger, quicker fighter. Within our system, there are specific Krav Maga drills and specific Trojan workout strength and conditioning drills. It was during my four-year tenure at the university in Haarlem that I developed these early workouts. I still do this one when I don't have much time.

10-MINUTE DRILL

- Set the audio timer so that it beeps loudly every 60-seconds.
- "Hardstyle" plank for 10 seconds
- Swings, between 12-20, depending on my mental state (MEIS)
- Rest till the next beep, repeat 10 times.

I would do this drill five times a week, raising the intensity each session. The duration, ten minutes, stays the same. You attempt to jack up the intensity. How? More swings! Another way to ramp up intensity is to reduce the rest periods. I would challenge myself to do one more swing per workout. The workload increases while the resting time shortens. If I could do 14 swings per minute and could finish the workout with clean technique, I would strive to do 15 in the next session. My goal was to do 20 swings per minute. When I could, I would shift to the next heavier bell and start the cycle over again.

You will find additional information about this section and for a guided workout at:

THE EMPEROR HAS NO CLOTHES

As a fitness professional, as a martial artist and as a lifelong athlete, I was perplexed, baffled and angry. In Holland the accepted orthodoxy for fitness was not working. Yet despite being practiced for decades and despite the fact that no one was making any progress using these outdated modes and methods, no one seemed to notice or care. I noticed and cared and now I had an alternate strategy. I had devised a method that would generate far better results in far less time.

When results are not forthcoming, real coaches makes changes and faux coaches make excuses. When you only have one way, one method, one protocol, fitness results might be forthcoming initially, but they will dry up quickly. Successful fitness is knowing what to do when results fade. Successful systems of fitness have built-in nuance and contrast. When results fade, the elite athlete has another radical protocol, ready to roll, ready to blast the complacent body out of its stagnation.

The orthodox fitness protocol routinely prescribed consisted of 30-40 minutes of cardiovascular exercise, usually done on an aerobic device, perhaps a stationary bike or the treadmill. The cardio was complemented with a "strength" program, consisting of a series of progressive resistance isolation exercises done on techno gym machines.

This approach to exercise and fitness was widely accepted and used without question. The results were decidedly underwhelming—but no one seemed to notice or care. I felt like the little boy in the Hans Christian Anderson fairy tale that blurts out the obvious: The Emperor has no clothes, or, in this instance, the classical fitness approach has no results!

I wanted to compete against the classical fitness approach in some sort of test or study. I knew that if I could create some sort of head-to-head challenge, the Trojan Workout would out-perform and out-deliver results derived from any orthodox fitness system. Since no such challenge or study existed, I set about creating one.

My goal was to twofold: yes, make students stronger and fitter, but also do it in far less time. I had been exposed to the classic orthodox approach to exercise and fitness (the orthodox dietary prescriptions are equally flawed) for many years. My observation was the exercise intensities were insufficiently intense to generate physiological results. In the effort to make exercise "safe" the controlling experts emasculated the effort.

The experts thought that by reducing the intensity, the sheer physical effort, and by compensating with more training volume, the results would come out the same. There is no adaptive response by the body if there is insufficient effort. Why would performance improve or the physique improve in response to sub-maximum effort? What is needed is herculean effort. With supreme effort, we can achieve more with less: superior results with less training time. Effort, hard, dedicated effort, is what creates results and powers the Trojan Workout.

People were uniformly using the orthodox training strategies and uniformly not obtaining results. People were wasting time in the gym and getting nothing in return. I knew I could get dramatic results for anyone that used the Trojan Workout with the requisite intensities. I knew my way around at this point, so to get my test off center, I gathered together a group of students from the university. I made sure none were star athletes and none had ever done the Trojan Workout. That was essential, my main criteria, my particular goal was to attain extraordinary results for ordinary people. My research question was postulated and predicated thusly...

- Create a test sample group of untrained individuals
- Divide participants into two subgroups
- Half of participants will use orthodox fitness modes
- Half of participants will exclusively use the Trojan Workout
- Establish an agreed upon series of testing benchmarks.

How does the training effect of the Trojan Workout differ from a regular Fitness Workout in an eight-week training period?

THE RESEARCH SUMMARY: the aim of this research is to compare the effectiveness of Trojan Workout against a regular fitness workout, during a training period of eight weeks. Effectiveness is understood to be the development of conditioning, for both power and endurance.

Forty subjects performed a fitness test (average age: 25 years, average height: 172 cm, weight 72.4). The fitness test was based on the YMCA test set and consisted of the long jump test, push-up test, pull-up test, sit-up test and the shuttle run test.

In addition, a questionnaire has been completed. Based on the results, the subjects were matched and divided over the Trojan Workout group or the Fitness group. Both groups trained twice a week.

The Trojan group did interval training at high intensity, mainly with kettlebells. The training lasted a maximum of 30 minutes.

The fitness group trained with a standard fitness schedule that met the guidelines of both "Fitvak" and ACSM. The training consisted of strength exercises on machines in which all major muscle groups are addressed, followed by a cardio program of 3 x 12 minutes.

The results of the fitness tests were assessed on the basis of already available and reliable reference tables, taking into account age and gender. On the basis of this, a score was given per test, on a scale of 1 to 7. The average increase in score of the Trojan Workout was +1, while with the fitness group it was +0.75. It was striking that the growth was the same on strength, but on the conditioning part the Trojan showed growth, while the fitness did not. No significant differences were measured between the research groups, which is a consequence of a small sample.

When looking at effectiveness, it can be concluded that the Trojan Workout is a more effective way to improve conditioning. The Trojan Workout performed 8 hours of training at the end of the study, compared to 20 hours of training in the fitness group. To score 1 point higher on the YMCA score, 8 hours of Trojan Workout had to be done, compared with

21.5 hours of Fitness training. From this it can be concluded that for this research population the Trojan Workout gives an average 2.5x more effect than the Fitness workout.

Taking in consideration that the Trojan Workout group first needed to learn the kettlebell techniques that were used, like swings and presses with full body tension, this group took about 3 week (6 sessions) before people could start training effectively and intensively with safe form.

After the research, people that did Trojan Workout wanted to keep training. They were exited and felt like they got stronger. Many participants mentioned how they liked this new feeling of being strong. Most of the people from the fitness group that got the offer to train for free for the 8 weeks, didn't want to pay for future training, after the research was done.

THE RADICAL EXPERIMENT: THE TROJAN WORKOUT CHALLENGE

"...EMPOWERING ORDINARY PEOPLE TO DO EXTRAORDINARY THINGS."

By 2012 I felt that the concepts and precepts of the Trojan Workout were fully formed. While I was continually searching for new and better techniques, the structural architecture for the Trojan Workout had been arrived at. The philosophic guidelines and goals were established. I was free to juggle the component parts to create differing physiological effects while staying true to the characteristics that defined the Trojan Workout.

There was no doubt that the Trojan Workout had transformed my own physique and there was no doubt that this new brand of strength training was getting near instantaneous results for our growing army of students. I wanted to spread the word even wider about the incredible results being attained by everyone that used our new methodology.

I became super excited with my progress and was eager to see if I could replicate the fantastic results I was obtaining with others. I turned to my great friend Jan Hofman. Jan is extremely intelligent and a highly successful physical therapist. He became one of my first instructors in 2009. He assisted me in building Trainingscentrum Helena.

Together we traveled the world to participate in many different Kettlebell and bodyweight certifications. We were one of the first certified RKC instructors in the Netherlands. Jan is like a walking encyclopedia. In his behavior, he is a really modest guy; but he has an amazing amount of knowledge. I met him during my time teaching at the university where he was my colleague. We became friends and he started teaching at my gym. A few years later he started his own Krav Maga studio in his hometown Vlaardingen (near Rotterdam). I was honored that he asked me to use the name Trainingscentrum Helena for his own studio.

Jan was the first person outside of myself to use the Trojan Workout. Based on the outstanding results we obtained using the Trojan Workout, I decided to create a challenge. I have been accused of being an outside-the-box thinker and I felt that what was needed was some sort of outrageous yet doable challenge. I wanted a challenge that involved a large group. I wanted to have the Trojan Workout tested, in some sort of big event involving Trojan Workout students. What sort of challenge could the group achieve that would be truly sensational? I put my mind to creating some sort of herculean benchmark.

It was during this time that I first read about the latest fitness craze in a popular fitness magazine. It was another American athletic concept completely new to the Dutch audience: Urbanathlon. An obstacle course in the city. The Urbanathlon is a 12 kilometer run over and through a mix of obstacles, all the while running through the urban landscape. This sounded cool and caught my attention. This was not for the weak hearted.

What if you could cross-train regular people to be able to run, finish and do well in an Urbanathlon—but without training for it? My people would train, but the training would be confined to the Trojan Workout. No running and no practice dealing with obstacles.

My participants would not be elite athletes, these would be regular folks. Here was my idea: train thirty people; confine them to two Trojan Workouts per week. Nothing else. Would the Trojan Workout enable regular people to do something athletically demanding and totally outside their skill set?

I sincerely thought that this radical approach would work—but I had no way of knowing. I would limit everyone's training to two sessions per week, each session 30-minutes in length for a grand total of one cumulative hour of training per week training—nothing else! It was critical the thirty participants not engage in any other physical activity of any type or kind, otherwise the conclusions would be distorted and the results diluted.

What could be more impressive than having non-runners be able to cope with a 12-kilometer *obstacle course* run without any specialized training. There would be no running or practice dealing with the type and kind of obstacles they would encounter repeatedly, 25 times, during the 12-kilometer run.

I did not want serious runners to participate. I would not "stack the deck." I would purposefully seek out regular individuals; I was not seeking ex-athletes that could perform well and cast my system in a good light. Let the facts speak for themselves: I was strangely confident.

Would it not be sensational if 30 non-runners could successfully complete a 12-k obstacle course run—without having practiced any running or practicing overcoming obstacles?! To me, that would be mind-blowing: what a great endorsement for a system of strength. We would enable and empower ordinary people to do extraordinary things!

This would be an exciting experiment. It is only commonsense that if a person is training for a 12 K run to run as much as possible as far as possible and as often as possible. Further, if this is a 12 K *obstacle course* run, a military style event, commonsense would dictate to practice dealing with various obstacles.

My idea was to allow no running, no obstacle practice of any kind; the only training allowed would be Trojan Workouts and no more than twice a week for 30 minutes. I would not cherry pick elite athletes. My 30 participants would be regular folks. No walkers. I would insist on a two-hour time limit. I discussed the idea with some of my elite associates. To a person, they all thought this idea was absolutely crazy. Which only made me give it greater consideration.

Despite everyone's reservations I went ahead and created the Trojan Challenge. Within ten days I had my 30 participants, all of them screened and vetted. I had the cross-section of normal folks I sought. I had an even division between the genders and the ages were from a 19-year old to my oldest, a 59-year old man.

We set a challenge date. It allowed us 90-days to prepare. If we were purposefully limiting ourselves to two 30-minute sessions per week, then these sessions would need to be of the highest quality. I really stressed to those that agreed to participate that we needed to put 110% focus into every workout. If this was to succeed, those two thirty-minute Trojan Workout sessions needed to be intense, past all our previous efforts.

I focused on 'tactical' strength moves. To that end, I concentrated on heavy swings and snatches. Special emphasis was placed on tactical pull-ups and push-ups. Here are sample workouts we performed leading up to the Trojan Challenge...

Protocol

2x per week: Trojan Workout group session
1x per week: swing/ snatch protocol
4 times a week; a pyramid of 5-1 (Australian) pull-ups

Exercise: Pull-ups and snatches
Tools or mode: chin bar, kettlebell
Reps: every minute on the minute
Time: 30 minutes
Poundage: snatch size kettlebell

Swing protocol:
Perform an isometric plank for 10 seconds. Immediately perform 12 swings. Rest for the remainder of the timed one-minute period. Repeat this one-two-rest protocol every minute for 20-straight minutes.

Snatch protocol:
Perform an all-out set of snatches. Try to do as many technically correct reps as you can, in 1 minute. Then divide this number by 2 to decide your rep-range. Now you have your number of reps that you will do every 30 seconds. After every 30 seconds, you rest for 30 seconds. You try to do this for 30 minutes, so 60 rounds. After 4 weeks, you do an all-out set again to check if you can increase rep-range (the number of reps, divided by 2). If your rep-range is above 40 reps, you increase the weight of the kettlebell.

Pull-up protocol:
Practice your pull-ups daily, in a pyramid. Going from 5-1 reps, with enough rest in between so you won't fatigue or miss a rep.

The Trojan Challenge took place on October 31st in 2013. In addition to the 30 participants there was a sizeable crowd made up of husbands, wives, children, friends, gym members and supporters. The actual event was like a Sunday afternoon fitness festival. There was a palpable excitement in the crisp fall air as the contestants lined up at the start line. It was quite exciting when the start signal was given.

I ran along mid-pack, acting as a cheerleader and motivator—not that it was needed — these people were psyched out of their minds: the collective energy was off the chart; the cheer that went up when the gun went off sent a chill up my spine. The group was like a mob as it moved to and over and thru and under the 25 obstacles. Did they help each other? To some degree, but that team esprit was inspiring and thrilling.

Everyone made it. No one walked. Everyone finished before the two-hour time limit.

Wow!

The exhilaration was incredible. We all felt as if we had really accomplished something. I felt I had proved something. To myself and to the world. It is one thing to scheme and daydream—it is quite something else again to achieve that which you sought. Way back when this crazy idea formed in my head, had you asked me how many out of the 30 might actually finish, 100% would seem too good to be true—yet it was.

I spent a lot of time afterwards discussing the process and the event with the participants. The consensus was that the Trojan Workout prepared them well for the obstacles. More than one challenge runner indicated that without working hard on the Trojan Workout, there would have been no way for them to successfully negotiate the obstacles. Most were surprised at how well the high intensity Trojan Workouts positively affected their cardio capacity.

I worked the Challenge participants hard all through the process, and the closer to race day, the harder we worked. A lot of fitness types don't understand that the 'burst' or 'interval' cardio stresses we routinely apply during the Trojan Workout carries over into other athletic formats. The severe exertions we routinely subject ourselves to using the Trojan Workout protocols dramatically improves cardio conditioning. My feeling is that once you have acquired the type and kind of aerobic conditioning bestowed by the Trojan Workout, that quality of conditioning carries over in all types and kinds of athletic activity.

I noted when I was in the military spec ops that a lot of men that had excellent cardio condition only had this degree of aerobic excellence as long as they ran at a steady pace on relatively flat surfaces. Despite their ability to run a marathon, if you threw off their steady-state pace (like having to stop and exert extreme muscular effort to scale a wall or rapid-climb a rope ladder) they fell apart. As long as steady-state cardio adepts could exert in a measured way and at an even pace they could run or swim (or whatever) all day long.

But that is not life. Our Trojan Workout cardio conditioning is all about muscular exertions *placed in an aerobic format.* In a classical Trojan Workout intense muscular effort is interspersed with short rest periods and repeated every minute on the minute for 10-30 minutes. Our isometric strength—built and improved on through our planks and Trojan Pose—prepares trainees for the intense muscular exertions needed to scale a wall, leap a water hazard, or bound over a low wall. Our power is usable in every instance, our cardio is not conditional.

As you can see from the gallery of photos, this event was a smashing success in every way. The anticipation leading up to the event, the collective energy before during and after was indescribable and best of all, in the aftermath of the event everyone took their individual training to the next level; the event created an esprit de corps that I had only experienced in the military. The event was so successful, on every level and by every benchmark, that we ran the same event at the same time the following year—but that is another tale for another time.

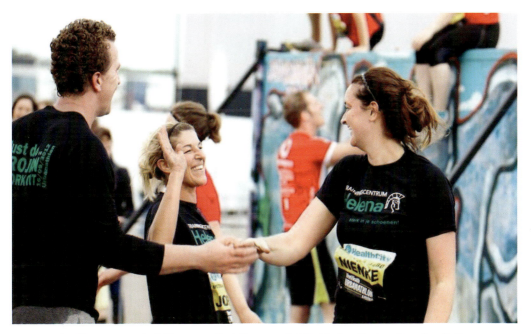

Everyone made it. No one walked. Everyone finished before the two-hour time limit.

SANDY

After the success of the two Trojan Challenges, after the success of Fitness Challenge, I began looking around for new ways in which to spread the word about the effectiveness of the Trojan Workout. It was tough to get attention. The fitness world was (and is) so crammed and jammed with options and possibilities that it makes it very hard for a truly effective method to cut through the bullshit.

I noted with a mixture of humor and disgust the proliferation of fraudulent fitness tools and fake methods being advertised on television. The craziness seemed to have no limit, no truthfulness or decency. Fitness tools and methods routinely make outrageous promises of amazing results with no sweat, no effort and no exertion.

"Obtain the body of your dreams with just two easy five-minute workouts per week. Build muscle and obtain the six-pack abs you have always wanted. And all in only fourteen days or triple your money back! But wait! Order now and receive absolutely free the Ab-Sizzler! Only three easy payments of $19.99." How does a legitimate tool and protocol compete for attention with outright lies?

I thought about who those mindless fitness ads were aimed at. These moronic tools with their impossible promises were aimed at the most unfit and uninformed portion of the population. Could I reach them? And, if they could, could these EZ fix types be coaxed into trying the Trojan Workout? Could the totally out-of-shape populace handle the Trojan Workout, in even its mildest form? If I could reach these people, could I offer them a tuned-down version of the Trojan Workout—yet still get outstanding results?

Now *that* seemed a worthy challenge.

I was more than a little hesitant to create some sort of 'Trojan-lite' for the pathetically unfit. Part of me thought, there should be a bare minimum, some entry level, below which you need not apply. That was a bit elitist, I decided.

What if I *could* create a version of the Trojan Workout, a version that could be used to help the most unfit? Rather than discard them, why not help them? Could I? I didn't really know. I had never worked with this segment before. Before I could work with them (I had decided I would) I had to reach them. But how?

Social media was the answer. I employed some out-of-character ads to attract attention. I was surprised with the positive response. Soon I was interviewing candidates and fine-tuning my tuned-down approach. Once I decided to work with the unfit, it began to dawn on me that this could be an important project. If I could obtain results for this discarded and ignored fitness population, the Trojan Workout could potentially 'break out' and garner some deserved widespread popularity. The users would be the winners.

Major auto makers like Porsche and Mercedes use their racing programs to develop the cutting-edge technology that eventually finds its way into passenger cars, making them more powerful and efficient. I would do something similar and take the hardcore Trojan Workout and make it user friendly to normal (or sub-normal) people. I would adapt and adopt and modify elite methods for those most in need.

The objective was to make the Trojan Workout doable for the unfit—but without losing its effectiveness. That is truly the razor's edge. If I made it too easy there would be no results. How do you train the untrained hard enough to obtain results—but without injuring them or hurting them? The untrained are truly delicate and too much too soon either hurts them or is so painful that they quit. The unfit are good at quitting fitness. They have a lot of practice.

Now that I had willing participants, how would I handle them? Unlike my studio students, these folks were non-athletes and would NOT be attending any of my classes. This would be remote coaching. We would stay in touch remotely. From a coaching perspective, everyone needed extra care and attention. No two were alike and they were all delicate snowflakes, as fragile as Faberge Eggs.

These people were not sturdy fit athletes, or even regular folks seeking to become leaner and fitter; these people were starting off below zero. These people were uniformly wobbly and un-athletic and the slightest over-exertion could cause them to rip or tear something—or could induce a heart attack.

Each person needed an individualized training program; I insisted on a face-to-face initial meeting. We would meet, go over the plan of attack; what was expected of them and what a commitment would entail. I was also sizing them up: if they were truly motivated, I could and would work with them. I had to weed out the insincere, the half-hearted or those without the life situation.

Often the client is ready and willing, but because of overwhelming time commitments cannot find the time or energy to fit fitness in. My unfit remote students needed to be willing and able to train; they needed to have a complementary situation. I was also looking for a little psychological grit or even a hint of desperation.

I worked with dozens of folks during this period, with varying degrees of success. One of our best examples was Sandy the bus driver.

Sandy stood five feet three inches and weighed 220 pounds. To be honest, initially I rejected her. She was too far gone, in my opinion. I didn't feel she had the burning desire. She tugged at my heartstrings when she broke down and cried upon learning I had rejected her. I relented on the promise that she would give it her best effort. And she did.

Working with Sandy required I develop some subtle psychological methods. She was an interesting case in that she did not respond to the standard enticements and motivations. She was convinced that she was beyond any kind of physical help and was therefore not motivated by promises of a transformed body. She was convinced that (genetically) she was cursed and prevented from any improvement or gain. She'd "tried everything" (highly doubtful) and "nothing worked."

Since she was immune to my usual exhortations. I decided to try a different approach. Rather than think of the Trojan Workout as some sort of body makeover fitness program, I told Sandy to think of the Trojan Workout as work. Work like getting up every damn day to drive the bus. Sandy was a damned good bus driver and while she might not believe she was capable of transforming physically, she knew how to get up and go to work and do the work and do the work faithfully and do it right.

I took away the bathroom scale. If this was going to be work, not transformational fitness, then I would eliminate the fitness report card, i.e. bodyweight reduction. In return for not being made to stand on the scale every week for another humiliating weigh in, Sandy would "just do the work." That became our motto, Just do the work… and do not worry about results. Do not worry about your bodyweight. Do not worry about the mirror. Just do the work. I knew that if she did the work the results would take care of the themselves.

Sandy was a good worker. Dutiful. Just like at work when she did something outstanding or got a written compliment from a passenger, she would get a commendation that would go into her bus driver permanent file. I attempted to replicate this by creating a spread sheet that chronicled her beneficial choices. When she passed on a candy bar or walked her groceries home she gave herself a happy face emoji on the spread sheet. When she did extra good on her nutrition, it was logged and passed on to me.

I became her boss at work and she responded well to this 'just do the work' approach. When we finally did break back out the bathroom scales she had lost 10 kilograms of body fat and muscled up nicely. That is when she really got traction.

Sandy was naturally stout, a compact woman with wide hips and thick bones. She took to strength training because of her body type and natural leverages. She became quite strong quite fast. I remember after one kettlebell workout where she out lifted a couple of the guys in the class. She beamed, "I like being strong!" she said in a typical understatement. She told me in private that one of the most satisfying moments of her adult life was when she beat her husband during a bicycle ride for the first time in her life. That was a miraculous event for her.

Because Sandy became strong quickly, she was able to maneuver her still-considerable bulk more easily, even while still big. Then, over time and with diligence, her body fat started melting away. They say that inside every fat person there is a thin person yearning to get out. Sandy discovered that underneath her blanket of fat was a powerful body. Nothing amplifies a person's enthusiasm like obtaining sensational results. To make a long story short, she lost 60 pounds in nine months. I would guess with a good degree of certainty that she also gained 5-8 pounds of muscle. This put her total fat loss at 65 to 68 pounds.

Can you imagine what that does for a person's self-image? Plus, Sandy was no spring chicken. Just shy of 40, she was a prime candidate for diabetes or heart problems. These sensational gains were obtained from a woman who was starting off standing in a hole, below zero.

Her first workout had to be limited to one set of three exercises. Sandy had a love for strong coffee—nothing wrong with that, assuming you don't load it up with sugar. Each time she made a pot of expresso I had her perform a farmer's walk with a light kettlebell, to and from the expresso machine. So, 3-4 times a day she would walk to and fro carrying her kettlebell.

In addition, several times a day I had her do a set of steep-incline pushups. This is a terrific, bench-press like exercise that gives the unfit all they can handle, yet in the safest possible way. They are so weak that even a slight incline will require an all-out effort from the out-of-shape. This is an excellent pectoral, deltoid, tricep and lat strengthener. If the unfit are unable to complete a rep, they simply stop and stand erect, ending the set. The third exercise I had Sandy do was the Trojan Pose. I showed Sandy how to lock down the isometric nature of the pose, when done right.

Each week I would slightly increase the duration of her exercise. In each of our three core movements, I would ask a bit more. Small incremental gains created compound interest; after the first month Sandy got traction in a way she'd never achieved before.

She turned another major corner when I suggested a dietary deterrent: I asked that she send me a phone photo of every meal and every drink she ate or drank. It seemed a strange request, yet it was a genius psychological stroke on my part. Sandy found the process had a self-regulating effect; she began to feel embarrassed sending me photos of ice cream sundaes or pie slices.

Rather than take the photo, she began not eating the bad stuff. She came to dread sending me an incriminating photo. I never said a word about it. I kept silent and never ever admonished her over any photo. She was honest to a fault and would never dream of cheating or not sending me the food photo after giving me her word. I told her I would never criticize, I would simply be the food photo repository.

In the first four-week phase, I introduced her to the movements, made her comfortable with the exercises, increased her strength and stamina and established a routine. We began a complementary nutritional program. In the second four-week phase, we strove for regularity: regularity in training and regularity with nutrition. When someone is as untrained and out-of-shape as Sandy was, gains are not the problem: avoiding injuries (the untrained are fragile) and staying consistent are the problem.

By the start of our third, four-week phase, Sandy had progressed to the point where she was "back to zero" and ready to start "real" training. She was no longer a delicate snowflake. Up until then everything had been remedial and designed to accommodate her frailty. After eight weeks of training under my remote supervision, she was no longer frail. She had already lost 10 kilos of body fat and added a significant amount of lean muscle. She felt so much better. Her quality of life went from awful to excellent in eight weeks. With her newfound strength she could power her bulk around with greater ease, making her quality of life so much better.

With her improved strength and cardio capacity Sandy now powered through her workday with a vim and vigor she'd never had before. Because of her inherent good-natured honesty, the self-reflective act of photographing food and drink worked: she cleaned up the food selections and reduced her portion size and cut back on her overall caloric volume and eventually got to the point where she was proud to send photos of the healthy foods she was selecting.

She held the course and improved in every way every day: her training poundage improved, her cardio capacity improved and her serious training, combined with her new relationship with food caused her to lose another 60 pounds of body fat while adding ten more pounds of muscle. She had a new lease on life.

She also changed me. Before this "challenged folks" undertaking, I had very little experience working with the feeble and unfit. I had avoided it and now I found I liked it. I liked the people. They were earnest, honest, mostly working class and most had bad habits (eating, smoking, drink, all of the above) that they had begun as teenagers. They were trusting but had low pain tolerance and no stamina. As a coach I was stimulated by the challenge: find techniques and ways in which to morph the out-of-shape into in-shape without damaging or hurting them.

At the end of eight weeks, Sandy was able to participate in the full-fledged Trojan Workout. It was, for me, inspiring. Sandy faithfully implemented our protocols. She exhibited tenacity and obtained results—it was extremely gratifying. Here were some of the written "tips" we devised; little mindfulness exercises, each designed to make her think about what she was doing instead of just mindlessly doing it... mindless eating is the very definition of nutritional habit force.

- When chewing a bite, don't be thinking about your next bite
- Sit when you eat
- Eat from a small plate (you will feel like you have more food)
- Chew your food well and chew mindfully—the opposite of absent-mindedly
- After every bite, put down your knife, fork or spoon

- When you want to eat something, ask yourself what it does for you
- Avoid industrial food that comes in a can and bag
- Read the recipe before you make it
- Decorate your plate like it is a piece of art
- When you eat, only eat: no phone, no television, feel free to chat with another human
- It's better to have big meals than a lot of snacks
- Start every meal with green vegetables
- Cheat as an exception: the best time to eat a cheat meal is after an intense workout

Here is snapshot of Sandy's Trojan Workout, one she would be capable of starting at week eight, after graduating four weeks of the introductory phase and four weeks of the more comprehensive phase.

Trojan-set
Trojan Pose — 10 seconds
Kettlebell deadlift/swing — 12 kilo kettlebell — 10 reps
Turkish Get-Up — plastic water bottle — 5 reps L/R

Between each Trojan-set: walk to the espresso machine and back, Farmer's Walk style, carrying the 12-kilo kettlebell in one hand. Switch hands on the return trip.

Perform this four-exercise sequence THREE times; rest 30-90 seconds between each cycle

Sandy would next perform the following three exercise sequence, three times...

Goblet squat — 12 kilo kettlebell
Wall push-up
Farmer's Walk to and from the coffee machine.

For the grand finale, Sandy would do a modified Tabata protocol. She would swing her 12-kilo bell as follows....

Session	Swings	rest period	number of cycles	
#1	20 seconds	30 seconds	six	50 second cycles
#2	20 seconds	30 seconds	eight	50 second cycles
#3	20 seconds	20 seconds	six	40 second cycles
#4	20 seconds	20 seconds	eight	40 second cycles
#5	20 seconds	10 seconds	six	30 second cycles
#6	20 seconds	10 seconds	eight	30 second cycles

I taught Sandy how to perform a safe swing using the Trojan Pose. I insisted she use full body tension in the forward part of the swing. I made sure she was doing a correct (and safe) hinge with her hips. This Tabata protocol improved Sandy's cardio capacity, melted off body fat and jacked up her sluggish metabolism. An amplified metabolism burns more calories, ideal for anyone intent on reducing body fat.

Sandy turned my philosophic "what if?" into concrete reality. My method helped an ordinary person with extraordinary tenacity to change their body and change their life. After Sandy, I knew our "tuned-down" Trojan Workout could dramatically benefit those that needed it the most. Sandy showed me that if the individual has the motivation and situation, our system works!

You will find additional information for this section and an effective workout timer at:

MONUMENTAL QUEST

DESPITE LIVING IN A MAELSTROM, I STILL MAKE TIME TO PURSUE MY OWN PATH

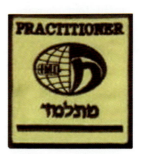

For six successive years I travelled to Israel. The center of the Krav Maga universe is in Israel. There are fifteen certified levels in Krav Maga. Proficiency is tested at each level. I would travel to either the International Krav Maga Federation headquarters near Tel Aviv, or alternatively to Expert Camp in Caesarea kibbutz Sdot Yam.

Practitioner

Grades P1 to P5 — student levels that form the majority of the Krav Maga community

P1 — a minimum of 45 hours, 4 to 5 months, 2 to 3 hours per week of training

P2 thru P5 — a minimum of 65 hours, 8 to 9 months, 2 to 3 hours per week of training

Graduate

Graduate Level: the student must master all skills in all P-level techniques. The majority of Krav Maga instructors are in possession of a Graduate level certification and are civil instructors. Krav Maga instructors are required to successfully complete the instructor training. Obtaining a Graduate level certification does not make you an instructor. The Graduate syllabus focuses on developing advanced self defense and fighting skills.

P5 to G5 — a minimum of 96 hours, a minimum time of one year between each level test

Expert

The elite of the elite: advanced security, law enforcement, close VIP protection and military techniques, hardcore sparring, subtle fighting skills are taught. Expert level Krav Maga practitioners teach other elite military divisions. Only a deserving select few achieve Krav Maga expert status.

G5 to Expert 1 — a minimum of one year

E1 to E2 — a minimum of two years

E2 to E3 — a minimum of three years

E3 to E4 — a minimum of four years

E4 to E5 — a minimum of five years

Over an eighteen-year period, I rose from Level 1 to Level 14. Level 14 is also called Expert Level 4. I was proud to attain the highest ranking ever achieved by a non-Israeli. The testing is insanely rigorous and becomes more so with each subsequent level. I had five months of concentrated training to prepare for my annual trip in 2017.

The certification testing lasts for five days and goes on from dawn till dark, all day, every day. As noted, the intensity level is directly proportional to the level; the demands for the higher-level certifications are light-years more severe and difficult than passing lower level certifications—not that any of them are easy.

Words cannot express the stress, mental and physical, that accompanies going through the certification process. The continual physical and psychological demands placed on you during the five-day certification process are never-ending and unrelenting.

Mobs were created and routinely assembled during the certification to create realistic crowd protection scenarios. At the level 13 certification, I was swarmed and run over, soccer thug-style, in a cert-staged riot. Have you ever wondered what it is like to be trampled by a stampeding mob? I can tell you from first-hand experience. I experienced it and survived; what does not kill us makes us stronger.

Krav Maga is not sport fighting. There are no rounds or referees or injury timeouts or rules. Krav Maga is combat fighting. All the things avoided and illegal in sport fighting are at the top of the street fighter's list of favored techniques—plus broken bottles, knives, clubs and guns. Remember, Krav Maga was originated by WWII Jewish resistance fighters battling roving bands of Nazi thugs—life or death stuff.

When you go to Israel and attempt to attain a higher Krav Maga ranking, they make it very hard on you because they take it very seriously. There is the eternal temptation to water-down or dilute a harsh, strict, effective method in order to make it more user-friendly and more attractive to the buying public. The Krav Maga powers-that-be, the keepers of the faith, insist that Krav Maga retain its realism and purity. No diluting, no watering down, no compromise: this is a combat fighting art without rules or restrictions. Realism rules. So expect to be subjected to realism. You are expected to react in accordance to the Krav Maga protocols.

Krav Maga is egalitarian in that anyone can use its core techniques and learn to defend themselves. "Stand up for yourself!" is a phrase I use repeatedly. It echoes my mother Helena's advice to "Stand strong in your shoes!" There is no way I will ever allow the dilution of the core Krav Maga techniques or principles.

SKILL TESTING

As instructed, I was driving around the Army base, traveling along a narrow street in a late model sedan. I was the driver and the beefy passenger next to me, a stranger, seemed nervous. There were two men in the back seat. The man sitting directly behind me was another stranger. I knew the older gentleman sitting in the right rear seat. I had noted the military tattoo on the left forearm of the stranger that sat behind me when he climbed into the car.

I drove carefully. We were traveling at 35 miles per hour. In the next instant, my burly, twitchy passenger whipped out a butterfly knife and placed it expertly on my carotid artery. I instinctively and without thought slammed the brakes on—hard. The knife and knife wielder were flung forward, as were the back-seat passengers. I immobilized his knife hand with my right hand and began pummeling his head with my left fist. I was hitting him hard and repeatedly, like a jackhammer.

By rising out of my seat (I'd unbuckled the seat belt) and pushing my bodyweight against his seat-belted body, I pinned him against the door. I got off three rapid shots, left hooks to his face. He was dazed. I slid both hands to pin his knife hand and began head-butting him.

When the knife fell out of his hand, I unbuckled his seat belt, pulled the door handle and pulled back as the passenger door opened. I shoulder- and elbow-jolted him until he fell out of the car onto the street. I slammed his door and sat back in my seat. I buckled my seatbelt and was about to burn rubber when the rear seat passenger leaned forward and wrapped my seatbelt around my neck. He yanked me backwards, hard.

In the split-second that it took for my head to impact the headrest, I turned my head and moved it sideways, finding a breathing space next to the headrest. This improvised Krav Maga maneuver ensured that my neck would not be broken and I would be able to breath.

I used my thumbs to release my neck from the belt. I slid my left arm through the space between the seatbelt and my upper body. Free, I flung myself knees first into the backseat. I was a millisecond away from unloading a straight right to the nose of my rear-seat attacker when the older passenger in the right seat said,

"Enough! Cease!"

The Krav Maga Master Trainer had seen enough. This had been just another drill done on just another day during my five-day Expert Level 4 Krav Maga certification.

Another day, a different drill. The scenario was blowing my mind. Which was exactly the plan. This specific drill was designed to test physical and mental ability to adapt. A big part of the Krav Maga certification process was the purposeful infliction of mental stress. Make no mistake about it, this five-day cert was voluntary boot camp and the mental abuse was as bad or worse than the physical abuse.

In this scenario we were assembled in the huge main gym. There was a riot going on. Literally, a mob of people fighting with one another. I was charged with handling a VIP and needed to be moved through the mob; I had to be super-aggressive protecting my civilians as I shepherded them across the room through the chaos. I really had to get physical with the "rioters." I pushed, shoved, punched and kicked my way through the mob.

I was immediately sent into a second room and told to deal with the situation. I walked in the room, still panting and recovering from battling my way through the rioters. Two women had ahold of each other's hair and were kicking and screaming. I had no earthly idea what I was walking in on. No one had prepped or alerted me. This was a test to see if psychologically I could "throw the switch" and morph from maximal animalistic brute force into low-key peacemaker all in an instant.

It took every bit of my self-control and willpower to make this dramatic psychological transformation. They were purposefully not listening to my low-key instruction to stop. I moved close to them and without screaming or being aggressive, I calmly grabbed one hair-puller's wrist and with a sharp, short jolt hit the back of her clenched fist with a single knuckle on my right hand, causing her to involuntarily open her fist full of hair. I instantly repeated the knuckle-on-fist technique on the second lady.

This little pressure point tactic would hurt like hell but would not leave a mark and the pain, though intense, was gone in an instant. In turn, each of the fighters would yelp, "Ow! That hurts!" as they let go, stood up and redirected their fury towards me. Inside of 15 seconds of entering the room, I had two very angry ladies now directing their anger towards me—and not each other—which was my exact intention. I must have passed the test, though no one at the time was forthcoming with any kind of post-drill critique or friendly approval.

I knew that my level Expert 4 certification test would be a living hell. I had already climbed the ladder from the first to the 13th level and knew that at every level the intensity and demands were kicked up a notch. My Expert Level 2 at Wingate Institute in 2011 had been hell. So I knew that this was going to be past all reasonable limits.

To prepare for the physical and mental abuse I was in for during the five days of the level Expert 4 certification process, I sought out professional help. I had four months to prepare. Mind you, I was working all day coaching and teaching classes and trying to have some semblance of a normal life. I could only apportion 10 additional hours per week for my pre-cert prep training. There are only so many hours in the day.

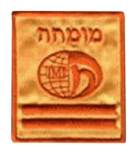

To prepare for the physical punishment I would be taking, I knew I needed to work on my "coping skills" under extreme pressure. In addition, I had to make sure my fighting skills were fine-tuned and at the highest level. In real world self-defense, fighting a lone opponent is one small aspect of the bigger self-defense picture. In real world self-defense there are weapons to contend with and weapons to use, there is fighting off multiple attackers and various escape and evasion situations.

I knew that part of my certification process would involve a drill that would require I fight 75 one-minute rounds, full-contact, with no rest in between. I would be fighting a series of fresh opponents. This would be a truly herculean feat and I worked hard knowing that I would soon be trying to stand and fight for 75 straight minutes—and who knew what exhausting drills would have already been done on that day. The 75 rounds of full contact would be just one of a half-dozen drills scheduled for that day.

I really needed work on my combat fighting skills. I wanted to be able to endure against many different fighting styles, many different body types and fighting strategies. I had to improve my ability to endure the grueling schedule. I had to work on my pain tolerance. I would be getting punched and kicked a lot over the five-day certification marathon.

In order to better absorb blows, you need to get punched and kicked. Without realistic, painful, limb-clashing blows and blocks, when you are barraged by them you wilt. I needed to be better able to be inflict damage. I needed to be better able to absorb punishment.

I knew just where to go and just who to enlist. I needed to have skilled fighters beat me up on a regular and ongoing basis. I needed to feel blows delivered by professionals. I needed to increase my ability to take a beating. But I had to do so while staying injury free.

I travelled to a famous MMA school in Amsterdam named R-Grip. I explained to the boys what was going on and that, essentially, I wanted to become a human punching bag. Once they understood that I was a serious person with real credentials and once they understood my mission they were more than willing to oblige.

Continuous sparing with people that know how to hit really hard is a fantastic way to improve your defensive fighting skills, pain tolerance and the ability to take a beating—assuming you can take it. I knew that I was going to be stressed for days on end physically and psychologically. The ability to endure and withstand extended periods of high-level physical and psychological stress is a requirement for passing level Expert 4.

I would travel to the MMA gym and spar with a never-ending succession of really good fighters. I was pushing past fatigue and learning to deal with very real pressure and very real pain. This strategy proved to be the perfect preparation.

After getting through it, after finishing the five-day marathon of torture, fighting, running, psychological stress, continual fatigue and pure pain, I looked back and thought—

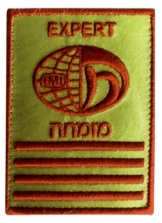

without all those hours doing Krav Maga drills with my instructors, without my Trojan Workout sessions and my sparring in the MMA gym for those four months prior—there was no way I could have lasted past day three.

It made all those early morning meditation and visualization drills, all those afternoon workouts, and all those nights of dragging my battered body home after being pummeled for hours on end by seasoned fighters seem worth it. The biggest honor of my life was being awarded the level Expert 4 certification. I had achieved the highest IKMF Krav Maga ranking ever by a non-Israeli.

THE FAST
SHIFTING MY METABOLISM FROM CARB-BURNING TO FAT-BURNING

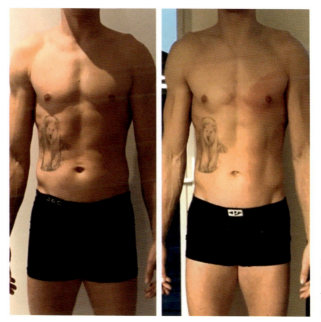

Before and after: melting off body fat to create a more efficient machine

As part of my preparation for my Krav Maga certification process, I knew that I needed to push both body and mind to the next level. I decided I would add a nutritional component to augment my preparation. I had been researching vigorously and decided I wanted to implement a fasting regimen.

While it might seem counterintuitive to starve oneself while prepping for an intense and prolonged event, such as the five-day certification process, handled right, I felt that a controlled fast would be the perfect kick-start for my prep process. I was not in bad shape, factually I was in fantastic shape—but I wanted to take my strength and conditioning into the stratosphere.

I liked the concept and philosophy of fasting, depravation. I felt I could use nutrition, the manipulation of calories and nutrients in such a way that physique and performance are taken to the next level. I also liked the idea of detoxing. Drain the body of all toxins, chemicals, impurities via the fast. Then, slowly, intelligently, precisely, add back food and drink.

I fasted for ten days. This fast wasn't about losing weight to look better or part of some spiritual journey; my motivation was purely athletic: lower body fat to improve stamina and endurance. I had come across some really exciting studies that showed how fasting and exercise could be combined to elicit dramatically improved endurance.

- Establish a 10 day fast protocol, with little to no food. And some specific supplements like omega 3
- Perform highly specific, aerobic exercise

I combined diligent fasting with repeated cardio. This protocol "teaches" the body to "hold" more oxygen in the blood. The fast eliminates insulin secretions and shifts the body from sugar-burning mode to fat-burning mode. Fasting starves the body of sugar, glycogen. The body, deprived of its favorite fuel, glycogen/sugar, will burn its second favored fuel: stored body fat. Fat fuel is twice as dense as carb fuel. A gram of fat contains 9 calories while carb calories are around 4 per gram.

In conjunction with the ten-days fast, I would start my day off with a run. The goal was to establish the optimal pace for my 30-minute morning runs. At the end of the ten-days fast I had sliced running the same distance from 30-minutes to 22-minutes, this while maintaining the same heart rate. I performed dramatically better with no more exertion.

Since a single certification test could take upwards of eight hours to complete, improving physiological efficiency was paramount. By every benchmark my counterintuitive inclusion of fasting worked past expectations.

POST-CERTIFICATION DE-BRIEF

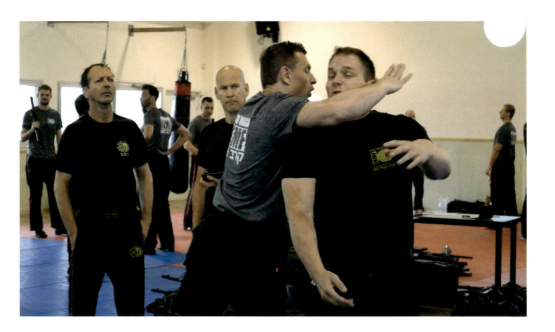

Looking back and looking ahead

In January 2017 I got the message that I would be allowed to participate in the Expert 4 exam of the IKMF. What a challenge! I would be the first Dutch person to participate in this exam. I wanted to use the opportunity to increase the pressure on myself. All eyes would be on me. I would inspire others.

I ask a lot of myself because I believe that by putting oneself on the spot you create a mindset that brings about growth. That does not mean that everything went smoothly. The day before my exam I had pangs of anxiety and I suffered from increased levels of stress. I felt a duty to my followers to succeed. I felt the pressure of performance and I realized I could fail and embarrass myself.

The evening before my exam I got the message that I had to do my Expert 3 exam again. On the morning of my exam the instructor put a real pistol in my hand instead of a practice weapon. "Show me that you can get along with it." He said.

I am no stranger to firearms. The first thing I did was check if the weapon was loaded. Even though I knew for certain that the weapon, a Glock 9mm, was not loaded, I deliberately and purposefully pulled the trigger as I aimed at the attackers during my exam. I found this was something uncomfortable.

The exam went by fast. It was like standing five feet from a passing freight train, it happened in a blur. Because I was the only one tested for level 14, I was tested non-stop under the critical eye of Avi Moyal, Master and Chairman of the IKMF, and Israel Tamir, the boss of the Security and Law Enforcement Krav Maga division.

I usually had to perform two repetitions of a particular technique then immediately move on the next technique. This went on non-stop for an hour in 90-degree heat. Over the course of a typical day we were allowed ten second breaks to drink water once every two hours.

For one of my previous Expert level tests I had to fight multiple opponents. These were IDF soldiers wearing protective gear and going all out. Every minute for ten minutes I had to fight four fresh opponents without any break. By the end I was so tired I missed blocking a high kick that hit my head so hard it burst my eardrum. At the time I didn't show any sign of the excruciating pain. Fighting four fresh opponents each minute for over ten minutes was pure hell.

Mentally, after the E4 exam my brain felt deep-fried. My E4 test was totally different from any other test. The big difference that the Level 4 exam was loaded with VIP security and Law Enforcement drills and Bodyguard techniques. When defending against knife attacks during the E4 exams, the instructor used tasers instead of real knives. If you wanted to avoid getting tasered, you had to be quick, light on your feet and completely in the moment. All in all, while I look back at the exam with pride, I am glad I am on the other side of it.

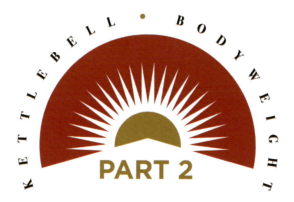

CONCEPTUAL BEGINNINGS

As a preteen, I was a reader of Greek and Roman mythology. There is something in these tales of Gods and warriors that appeals to young males and has for centuries. I read the mythological tales and became inspired by the heroic exploits of the mortals and they interacted with gods and demigods and vanquished beasts and foes and overcame obstacles as they went on quests and fought in wars. The Iliad and Odyssey and the tale of the Trojan War inspired me when I first read it. It inspires me to this day when I periodically reread Homer's epic.

The siege and fall of Troy ("Beware Greeks bearing gifts") was, for me, the most moving and inspirational tale of all. Most people would mistakenly think I was a fan of the Spartan approach: the warrior race, the stand of the 300, the Sparta lifestyle and mindset. Factually I was far more attuned to the Trojan philosophy of life and living.

In many ways, the Spartans were a death cult. The harshness, cruelty, slaves and rigidity that defined them put me off. I felt that their culture was all about willpower, pain and unquestionable obedience to a rigid caste system. The Spartan society and mindset were the opposite of what I aspired to.

On the other hand, the Trojan culture seemed the complete opposite. Trojan society was enlightened and placed a premium on knowledge and learning. Trojans sought out innovation. They didn't own slaves. Trojans valued innovation over conformity and sought to expand and improve all aspects of their society.

While the Spartans depended on willpower and tenacity the Trojans depended on intelligence and enlightenment. While the Spartans looked suspiciously at any deviation from their iron methods, the Trojans welcomed and encouraged innovation. The Trojan approach inspired me and shaped me. As a boy reading about heroic Trojan role models, I formed my desire to become a fighter and a soldier.

I gave a lot of thought to my underlying strength philosophy. I needed a phrase that captured and identified this new approach to strength training, something that would encapsulate and differentiate my protocol from the rest of the herd.

"Trojan" kept pushing its way into my head.

There were all kinds of subtle and overt clues: my mother was named Helena, as in Helena of Troy. Helena, the most beautiful woman in the world, the feminine ideal, strong mentally and physically. Now a man with a beloved mother named Helena is naturally inclined towards all things Trojan. The phrase "Trojan Workout" instantly resonated with me. It felt right.

Once I labeled my new comprehensive strength strategy the Trojan Workout, the workout seemed to redefine itself, almost as if it had a mind of its own.

PHILOSOPHIC UNDERPINNINGS

The goal of the Trojan workout is to maximize usable athletic strength across the entire strength bandwidth. Follow the protocols of the Trojan Workout with great precision and exactitude and reap truly profound benefits on a multitude of levels...

- **Power and strength:** exponentially increase these premier bio-motor attributes
- **Longevity:** retain function and athletic ability late in life and do Trojan Workout for the rest of your life
- **Sustained power output:** obtain strength and feel strong
- **Lean muscle mass:** increase muscle mass, increase muscular horsepower
- **Efficient:** no need to live in the gym, short intense sessions, optimal time efficiency
- **Improve body composition:** coordinate with sensible nutrition and get ripped
- **Improve heath:** a leaner, stronger, fitter person personifies vibrant health
- **Resilience:** improved ability to absorb punishment and bounce back from injury
- **Improve confidence:** improved by progress and growing power
- **Accessible to all levels:** everyone uses the same training templates, what varies is the intensities
- **Fun:** never the same, variety makes training challenging and appealing, never a dull moment
- **Safety:** maximum effect with minimum risk of injuries

We could go on but that's a good start. There are highly specific protocols that need to be followed. There is a totality about the Trojan Workout. There are many moving parts that are designed to interact in a certain way. It is important to implement the Trojan Workout in its totality; do not pick and choose. It all fits together seamlessly. Do not dissect the Trojan workout; use it as was intended and reap optimal benefits. All levels use the same template. Regardless if you are an elite athlete or an out-of-shape business executive, the drills and protocols are the same; what changes is the intensities and payloads.

THE PSYCHOLOGY OF THE TRUE TROJAN

THE PAYOFF IS ENJOYMENT OF THE PROCESS, NOT IN ARRIVING AT SOME MYTHICAL FINAL DESTINATION

Modern fitness is motivated by vanity. Look better, develop a six-pack set of abdominals, get fit for the beach or the mountain lake; everything is dependent on other people's *visual impressions* of your body. The modern fitness devotee seeks the approval of others. Approve my body, gaze at me and not be repulsed. Optimally my body is so sensational I am envied for my physique and desired sexually. It is no surprise that vanity fitness uses bodybuilding protocols. Vanity fitness is all about achieving, attaining, and arriving at that final physical destination, the perfect body you have always wanted and craved. Form over function.

Obviously, this is the exact opposite of what our philosophy is all about. Our approach is all about *function*. When the athlete improves their functionality in the various drills, form—the human body—automatically improves. This as a side benefit to becoming stronger, fitter, more agile and vital. By improving Trojan Workout performance each successive week, for weeks on end, the body improves, it becomes dramatically stronger.

The Trojan Workout creates lean, athletically functional muscle and by becoming dramatically fitter, the athlete burns off body fat. Best of all, the morphing of the body occurs naturally, as a direct result of improving the five bio-motor attributes: speed, strength, endurance, flexibility and agility.

In addition to working the five interrelated physiological elements, there is also an overarching *psychological* element. The Trojan psychology is very real and very well thought out. My own psychological journey, my mental evolution began as the bullied preteen. From this fear space, I compensated by taking up martial arts. Psychologically, I discovered very early on that I had the ability to immerse myself, to lose myself, in hard and intense physical training. I had a highly developed mindset heading into the special forces. My military training melded perfectly with my martial mentality.

Psychologically, it all came together when I began my Krav Maga immersion. The Krav Maga community had a long tradition of psychological emphasis, long before I began my Krav Maga journey, now two decades ago. In Krav Maga, control of the mind, willpower, pain tolerance, the ability to endure, stress control and purposeful aggression are identified and trained. Krav Maga placed great emphasis on developing the mental characteristics that are common to elite fighters and warriors.

The Mind can be the athlete's best friend or worst enemy. Over the years (decades, actually) I have developed a highly evolved and highly effective psychological approach designed to improve results derived from the Trojan Workout. A focused and concentrated mind takes training performance to the next level. Conversely, a distracted or preoccupied mindset degrades reflexes, technique and performance. I have developed drills and protocols aimed at improving psychological performance to improve physiological performance.

What a truly amazing thing to be able to improve the quality of the workout, strictly through mental recalibration. When you look a little deeper, psychologically, the ideal Trojan Workout mindset is clear, open and alert, without preoccupation or daydreaming; present and in the moment. This is a learned skill. It takes time, attention, diligence and patience to morph the mind.

I ask the students that train with me to become hyper-alert the instant they enter my training center for their Trojan Workout. As soon as my students pass through the door and into my gym, I ask them to adopt a Krav Maga mindset (Krav Mindset) and take in everything they see upon entering: the people, the room, the lights, the details.

Why do I ask them to do this, i.e., engage in an awareness drill prior to a Trojan Workout? The act of intense observation will automatically quiet an overactive brain. By trying to take in small details, their attention shifts from inward, from mindless mental chatter, to outward focus. By retaining this psychological shift as they prepare for the actual workout, they attain a mentally quiet, receptive mindset, the perfect mindset for an intense Trojan Workout.

This is one of many mental awareness tactics I expropriated from Krav Maga. You cannot absorb sensory input if you are preoccupied, distracted or daydreaming. Preoccupation is the enemy of perception: to see, to *really* see, you need be mentally quiet, alert and absorbing. During the actual workout, performance is exponentially improved if the trainee adopts a "controlled frenzy" approach. Optimally, I want trainees engaged and aggressive; the focused athlete obtains the most out of the Trojan Workout.

Another of my favorite mental drills is what could be slow-motion concentration drills. The procedure is quite simple: pick a movement, an exercise, perhaps a right cross or a Turkish Get-up. The mental aspect is in the performing: I might ask that the trainee take five full minutes to complete a Turkish get-up. No, that is not a typo, five minutes for a single movement. Why? If you lose concentration for an instant the pose immediately disintegrates. This slow-motion drill is almost a pantomime and acts as a concentration builder.

I myself will use the slow movements as a form of meditation; we breathe and move slow and precise, the goal being to not lose concentration for a single instant. Another awareness drill I use and recommend involves intense focus on a small object, a candle flame, a red dot on a white wall... sit quiet, settle into rhythmic breathing and do not let the eyes wander from the object or spot. Avoid mindless mental chatter. Focus like a laser. This one pointed concentration has many practical applications. What I and others have found is that mindfulness maintained during training not only improves workout performance, it also reduces injuries and accelerates recovery.

COMPETE WITH YOURSELF! LEARN TO LOVE THE PROCESS!

We compete with ourselves, not with one another. The goal is to improve on the current version of who we are—exalted or diminished—wherever we are at, whoever we are, currently, so we can improve upon what we are. This idea—compete with yourself, seek to improve on who and what you are—will, over time morph a negative self-image into a positive one.

Success changes a person. The small, consistent gains made consistently using the Trojan Workout generates enthusiasm. We become genuinely enthused about our results and this makes us want to redouble our efforts. By learning to love the process, continual adherence is assured.

If a person is in love with a goal, particularly a vanity goal, when they achieve that goal—now what? There is an old cliché, 'be careful what you wish for, you might get it.' Nowhere is that truthful cliché more appropriate than in the pursuit of vanity fitness.

When psychology is used to fall in love with the process, the battle is all but won. Real fitness, true fitness, functional fitness finds joy in the process. True fitness is a process, not an event.

COPING WITH FATIGUE

The Trojan Workout is not about avoiding fatigue, the Trojan Workout is all about embracing fatigue, understanding that every Trojan Workout SHOULD induce fatigue. The way in which to learn how best to deal with fatigue—to overcome fatigue and to extend our fatigue limits and capacities—is to continually deal with it.

How you deal with fatigue during your Trojan Workouts is extremely important. Our Trojan Workouts are, by design, short and intense. The dilemma is to deal with fatigue without it degrading our techniques. Injuries occur when technique breaks down. The ideal Trojan Workout takes the trainee deep into the fatigue zone—but safely and without technical degradation.

One fatigue-fighting strategy that I developed was to insist all students begin and end the training session with an all-out Trojan Pose. Assume the stance, assume the position, begin the systematic increase of isometric muscle tension: each time you hit the Trojan Pose you need to seek to exert harder, deeper, tensing all the way down into your bone marrow.

Using the Trojan Pose to commence a workout is an ideal way in which to transition from civilian mindset into warrior mindset. Using the Trojan Pose to finish a workout is you telling your body and showing yourself that despite deep and real fatigue, you still have more left. You always have more. However, this is a learned skill. It is only after actually performing an all-out Trojan Pose at the end of an all-out, fatigue-inducing Trojan Workout that you understand the post-pose exhilaration.

In Krav Maga it is taught to never show fatigue. Doing so would create an opportunity for an opponent or a predator to strike. When a violent criminal senses weakness, any outward fatigue, any obvious signs of physical exhaustion, this is perceived as a signal to attack. In Krav Maga we perform drills that feign normalcy when we are factually exhausted.

I advise my Trojan Workout trainees to do likewise: avoid obvious signs of fatigue or exhaustion. Carry yourself with control and dignity. Do not allow yourself to show fatigue. Make a point of pride. Stand strong in your shoes.

Fatigue can be thought of as a mental barrier. One that should be overcome. Hide the fact that you are tired. Be an actor. If, in a street fight or during a conflict, you let others see that you are tired, you will look like a weak victim. Predators sniff out weakness and pounce. It takes mental strength to stand straight when exhausted. Do not show that you are tired. Ever.

PUT IN THE WORK

Competing with yourself is a concept that is central to the Trojan philosophy. The idea behind the concept is to stop comparing yourself to others. Compete with yourself. This way you are self-contained and never without a goal. The goal is the same and eternal: improve thy self.

Mainstream fitness experts champion shortsighted "status" goals. Get in shape for the beach, lose weight for the class reunion, get lean to fit into the wedding dress, lose weight, look better, obtain six-pack abs, get ripped... all are appeals to our vanity. The status goal is dependent on the opinions of others, you are not dieting and doing crunches to impress yourself, you are striving for a six-pack to impress others. You seek approval, you seek being envied and desired.

The Trojan Workout strives for something different and something quite profound: the Trojan Workout goal is about improving only you. Wherever you find yourself, fit or unfit, regardless, with regular and repeated practice of the Trojan Workout you will improve all aspects of your physical self. And in doing so automatically improve all aspects of your psychological self.

Those that adhere to the principles and tenants of the Trojan Workout will undergo undeniable physical and psychological progress. Diligent adherence to the tenants of the Trojan Philosophy is based on the idea of "just putting in the work—and without expectation." This is fitness Zen in the purest sense.

Those that 'just' put in the work and do so with the appropriate diligence and the appropriate intensities undergo profound physical and psychological changes: they become empowered as they improve strength, speed, endurance, flexibility and agility. By improving the physical, by putting in the work, the psychological well-being automatically improves.

There is an inherent danger with status goals in that once the goal is attained, retaining becomes difficult if not impossible—why? The process used to attain the status goal is unsustainable as a lifestyle. Too restrictive, too severe, too unhealthy to be sustainable. The Trojan Workout offers a viable alternative: by just putting in the work you obtain the results using a sustainable lifestyle.

The term self-esteem has become a bit of a politically correct phrase, having a positive self-image breeds confidence and confidence creates calmness and centeredness. Confidence depends on the situation. In any situation you can learn how to become more confident. It's a mental skill.

Part of the Trojan Workout physiological philosophy is aimed at developing the ability to predict feelings. If you are able to predict your feelings, then you can better control your feelings. What do we mean by 'predicting feelings?' Predicting feelings could also be described as knowing how you are going to feel before an event occurs. This develops into a sixth sense that puts you into a state of control. When you are in control of a situation you are rewarded with self confidence.

Preplanning predicts feelings. Mentally construct your next move and you successfully predict an about-to-happen feeling. Preplanning creates self-fulfilling prophesies. What can we control, physiologically? One thing in our control is adherence to training. First and foremost, we must show up. You can control that. If you show up to work out you can then control the degree of effort exerted during the training session.

THE MENTAL EFFORT INTENSITY SCALE (MEIS)

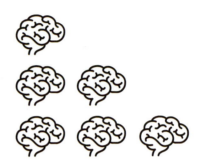

One of the unique qualities of the Trojan Workout is the purposeful modulating of training intensities. I devised the Mental Effort Intensity Scale as a way to quantify the degree of mental effort used to complete a drill or protocol. A simple 1 to 3 numeric scale is used to determine the degree of mental effort required or expended.

How to determine the appropriate MEIS for any workout

- Make adjustments based on life's realities
- If circumstances are not favorable, reduce the intensity
- If circumstances are favorable, increase the intensity
- The use of differing intensities is rewarding and recommended
- MEIS is used as inducement: rather than skipping a workout, reduce the MEIS

Warm-ups always provide feedback. Even if you have already set your MEIS for this workout, you can still make some adjustments. Listen to your body and make smart decisions. Sometimes, you feel good—yet still are not performing at your best. Lower the weights, change the work-rest ratio or skip an exercise in your program.

My friend Lucia Rijker was one of the best female fighters the world. She was scheduled to fight the main event in Mandalay Bay, Las Vegas against Christy Martin in an epic fight. On the last workout before the fight she told me later, she wasn't herself, she felt 'off.' Her trainer insisted that she had to do this final hard work-out. "I should have listened to my own feelings" she said. During the workout she tore her Achilles tendon and would never fight again.

Mental Effort Intensity Scale (MEIS Guidelines)

The higher the MEIS number the greater the degree of difficulty. The greater the degree of difficulty, the more mental focus and effort are required. How does an athlete determine their proper MEIS? Here are a few guidelines...

Complexity: sometimes low-intensity workouts are precisely what is needed. One way to create a less intense workout is to select simpler exercises, less complex movements. A swing would be considered a simple movement while a snatch is far more complex and requires far more attention, focus and motor-skills. A pistol is more challenging than a conventional squat. A Turkish get-up is far more complex than a kettlebell press. Reduce the complexity of the exercises and lower the MEIS.

Another way to modulate the complexity is to create shorter exercise "links" in your Trojan Set. A complex sequence could consist of a plank followed by push-ups, snatch, wall jumps and ending with bear crawls. A more simplistic format of lesser complexity would be swings followed by squats.

Intensity: modulate intensities upward or downward, depending on what is appropriate. To increase workout intensity, extend the duration of the session (within 30 minutes), increase the pace, add to the payloads, increase the number of sets and reps, alter the techniques. Modulate intensity by improving or disadvantaging leverage. Don't forget symmetrical and asymmetrical exercises: make it easier by doing pushups with two hands and make it harder by doing them with one.

Comfort: another way to modulate MEIS is to perform exercises that are more comfortable for you. We all have our exercise preferences, our likes and dislikes. Make it easier on yourself by selecting a familiar favored exercise and perform it in a favored way. Conversely, when the comfort level needs to be decreased, simply select a movement you do not particularly care for and perform it with great concentrated effort. Easy familiarity lowers the MEIS while complexity and difficulty increase the MEIS rating.

KEEP A POSITIVE MENTAL ATTITUDE (PMA)

Perception is everything. I have in the past studied with and under many excellent coaches, and some really bad ones. Sometimes I think I learned as much from the bad coaches as I did from the good ones. One common trait amongst my bad coaches was they all created a negative training environment. Because of my experiences with negative attitudes, I am determined to create a positive mental attitude (PMA) in every Trojan Workout training session. Just as negativity is infectious, so too is PMA.

A workout done with a positive attitude enables you to dig deeper, train harder, go longer. Fear and anxiety thrive in a negative atmosphere. PMA is like brilliant sunlight let in on a darkened room. Anxiety and fear adversely affect performance whereas a PMA allows the trainee or warrior to get psyched up in the best possible way. When we are enthused we tear into our workouts and do so with a fervor totally lacking in a negative, prison camp-like training environment.

Real confidence, true confidence, not fake or pretend, is built as a result of diligent practice and extreme effort done over a protracted period of time. Success breeds success: by compiling an uninterrupted series of excellent Trojan Workouts, body and Mind are transformed. This is best accomplished in a positive, uplifting workout environment.

Habit-force, force of habit, is real: there are good habits and bad habits. A good habit is an action or deed that creates a positive outcome; a bad habit is an action or deed that negatively impacts Mind or body. Obviously, over time, the smart individual seeks to replace bad habits with good ones.

One example of replacing a bad habit with a good habit is training related. It is very fashionable in mainstream fitness, HIT and bodybuilding, to perform an exercise "until failure." I consider this a bad habit for several reasons: going to failure is always preceded by a disintegration of technique; when technique breaks down is when injuries occur. In addition, from a psychological standpoint. I want all Trojan Workouts to end as a success, not a failure. I want the trainee to triumph and feel triumphant. This is hard to do when you have just beaten yourself into the ground performing a very dangerous exercise in a very fatigued and sloppy fashion.

You will find additional information for this section and about the mental power principles at:

Successful athletes develop incredible "muscle memory" and once they possess the muscle memory, they never entirely lose it. It might lay dormant for years, but given the right stimuli, the correct exercise dose at the requisite intensity and muscle memory will come alive. Basketball hall of fame player Steve Nash once spoke of his mental preparation for shooting foul shots from the free-throw line, "Before every foul shot, I think of the thousands of successful free-throws I have made over the years." Talk about PMA!

Trojan Exercises

Always ok	Sometimes	Never
Swing	Push press	Sit-up
Squat	Running	Burpee
Clean	Endurance plank	Biceps curl
Press	Mountain climbers	Triceps extensions
Push up		Kipping pull-ups
Pull up		
Hardstyle plank		
Isometric holds		

THE TROJAN WORKOUT VERSUS RUNNING

Don't get me wrong—I have nothing against running. I ran everywhere as a young martial artist and I ran all the time in the military. Handled right, running is a fine skill and will provide the diligent runner with stamina, endurance and, if coordinated with a sensible nutritional program, a reduction of body fat. However, too much of a good thing can be a bad thing. What attributes are obtained by running?

First and foremost, the diligent runner obtains cardiovascular fitness. The internal organs are stimulated, they are flushed with blood and oxygen, they are accelerated and strengthened. Running stimulates the heart, causing it to send blood coursing through the veins and arteries. When organs are stressed, systematically, they strengthen and grow in response to the stimuli. On the downside, running taken to an extreme, can create repetitive motion injuries, shin splints and chronic knee and ankle stress. Heavy people that are made to jog on concrete sidewalks routinely suffer from impact injuries and repetitive motion induced stresses.

Too many runners just run. As a sole source of exercise, running is one-dimensional and inefficient. Even limited to cardio, running is deficient in that it only uses two limbs, the legs, to generate 100% of the cardio effort. In the Trojan Workout all four limbs, arms and legs, are used to generate a much deeper and effective training inroad. The solution most runners apply to becoming fitter is more running. This is a bad idea. Available training time should always include strength training.

Is there a way to replicate the benefits of running without the drawbacks?

The whole point of the Trojan Challenge was to show that non-runners that engaged in the Trojan Workout could obtain all the attributes needed to run—without running. The expert use of a kettlebell can replicate and exceed the cardiovascular stresses associated with running. Want to accelerate the heart rate? Use the tools and modes we use in the Trojan Workout. Want to send blood coursing through veins and arteries? Use the tools and modes of the Trojan Workout. Want to strengthen internal organs and burn off body fat? Use the Trojan Workout.

THE TROJAN WORKOUT VERSUS HIGH INTENSITY TRAINING (HIT)

In my opinion, High Intensity Training (HIT) has been wildly successful on a worldwide basis because it stands in stark contrast to conventional fitness taught at conventional fitness facilities. The orthodox gym template is to create a spacious facility that houses an armada of exercise machines... progressive resistance machines of every type and kind, all dedicated to isolation exercises. In addition, an armada of aerobic machines of every type and kind is required, usually leg-only.

The personal trainers working at these conventional fitness facilities are schooled in bodybuilding strategies all aimed at vanity goals. HIT training positioned itself as exactly opposite: no lifting machines, no cardio machines, no personal trainers preaching bodybuilding. Instead, HIT training made a lack of that stuff and raw tools a selling point. This wasn't shallow vanity pursuits using super-expensive devices, this was barbells, ropes, kettlebells, chin bars and running. This wasn't about vanity. HIT was about function and improving athletic ability.

On the downside, because of the vast array of exercises taught, not all the exercise got taught with the subtlety required. I also strongly disagree with the promotion of competition amongst members. In my world we compete against ourselves, not each other. When speed and status goals are stressed, quality technique goes flying out the window.

It is my contention that diligent and appropriate practice of the Trojan Workout can replicate the functional results derived from the HIT training protocols. If the final desired result is to develop athletic function, and all that goes with it: strength, speed, endurance, flexibility and agility, then the Trojan Workout delivers on all counts.

Three thirty-minute Trojan Workouts per week will deliver maximum results for a minimal time investment—adding muscle and strength while improving stamina and endurance. If the Trojan Workout protocols are coordinated with a sensible diet, harmful and unhealthy body fat will be dissolved. A leaner more muscular you is a better you.

THE SEA SQUIRT

Why did evolution provide human beings with a brain? The brain's first function is to provide consciousness, awareness of who and what we are. The brain's second prime function is to enable the human body to perform adaptable and complex movements. Without movement, you have no impact on the world around you. Movement is how we interact.

Daniel Wolpert wrote an influential article for Ted.Com Talks entitled, "The Real Reason for brains." One of his illustrative examples is the tale of the lowly Sea Squirt. A Sea Squirt is a creature that lives at the bottom of the ocean. The Sea Squirt swims around in the ocean and at some point in its life, it attaches itself to a rock and never moves. Once the Sea Squirt attaches to a rock, that is it, the Sea Squirt will never move again.

From that moment on, the sea squirt gets the nutrient fuel needed for existence by eating its own brain. Because the Sea Squirt will never move again, the species determined that it could consume its own brain and still exist. The lack of any type or kind of movement makes thinking optional. If a creature can figure a way to exist without moving, there is no need for a brain.

I see a very real parallel between the Sea Squirt and our ever-more sedentary society. As a species, humans are attaching themselves to their office desks, to their sofas, beds and easy chairs much the same way the Sea Squirt attaches to a rock. So much of what modern man does can be done sitting or lying—computing, using phones, playing video games, watching shows or other visual entertainment.

Our species is morphing: our children learn to use their computer tablets before they learn how to talk. Even exercise is devalued; we drive from our air-conditioned office in our air-conditioned auto and arrive at an air-conditioned gym where we sit or lie down on various one-dimensional exercise machines. We can do one of three things on the fancy exercise machines: push, pull or pedal. We text between sets and never really sweat or strain.

Humanity could go the way of the Sea Squirt. As a species man uses the body less and less and when used it is used sub-maximally, using stunted forms of exercise. The old cliché is 'use it or lose it.' I sense that humanity is headed towards a Sea Squirt type of existence. Perhaps in 100 years (an eye-blink) humans will be amorphous blobs of soft flesh waited on by robots. Or perhaps our brains and consciousness will be housed in mobile machinery.

TROJAN WORKOUT GOAL SETTING

When new students express interest in learning more about the Trojan Workout and its precepts, I start off by telling them that the workout itself is a collection of principles, tools, methods, protocols, strategies and modes that are intermingled and intermixed in innovative ways designed to achieve highly personal goals.

Before we achieve anything of importance we must first define that thing; secondly, establish a goal, an ideal, benchmark; finally, use our broad array of strength strategies to achieve our highly defined and personalized goals. Once we have highly specified goals we create a timeline.

By working backwards from the goal, the Trojan Workout trainee is able to establish a realistic timeline, a week by week roadmap of sequential progress. One wonderful thing about strength training is that it is numeric, every training aspect and result has a numerical value, ergo the Trojan Workout is based on science, biology and objective logic.

We combine a grounding in science and logic with empiricism, actual results derived from implementing and following the Trojan workout. Our approach is always guided by results. How does the person new to our approach establish a goal?

Those that adhere to the guidelines of the Trojan Workout for ten to twelve weeks can realistically expect to also develop what I call the "Strong Trojan Presence," where a strong attitude is combined with a strong looking body and presented with proper posture and appearance. Change your physique and your life with ten to twelve weeks, 70 to 84 days of applied effort: three weekly training sessions, thirty minutes per session. If you do the math: over a 12-week cycle, 36 workouts would be performed. This equates to a grand total of eighteen cumulative hours of work—eighteen hours of work that will change your life.

You will find additional information for this section and effective goal setting at:

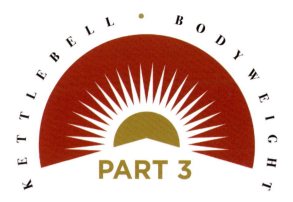

YOUR FIRST TROJAN WORKOUT...

At some point, after all the words are read, after all the thoughts are thought and all the dreams dreamed, it is time to turn thought into reality. You are ready to take your first Trojan Workout. The Trojan Workout uses a combination of kettlebell exercises and freehand exercises to attain the goal: make the trainee stronger, more muscular, far more fit and capable. This workout is designed to tax you, not break you.

One size does NOT fit all. While mainstream fitness trainers take great pleasure in beating the hell out of their hapless clients, the goal of the Trojan Workout is to coax gains, on a consistent and ongoing basis. Mainstream "no pain-no gain" types train everyone the same because they only know one way to train.

The Trojan Workout is, by comparison, subtle, nuanced and multileveled. The fantastic thing about the Trojan Workout is that an elite professional athlete can train alongside someone taking their very first Trojan Workout. How is this possible? While we all follow the same training template, graduations in intensity (payload) allow for everyone to participate. Everyone has three intensity options (variations) and a personal rep-range.

The goal of every workout is to gradually work up to current capacity. Only by seeking to safely and sanely equal and extend our current limits and capacities do we improve. No one magically gets fitter and stronger by doing the same things in the same way. There are a few tools needed before we start...

Kettlebell: I recommend a 16 kilo bell for men and a 12 kilo bell for women without kettlebell experience. Heavier bells can and should be used by stronger, fitter, more experienced trainees.

The floor: 2 square meters of obstacle free floor space. If you don't have a floor, you have bigger isues, as Al Kavadlo would say.

Chin-up/pull-up bar: in this particular sequence, access to a chin bar is required. If you are a home trainer, inexpensive doorway chin bars can be purchased.

Duration: all Trojan Workouts are limited to 30-minutes in length.

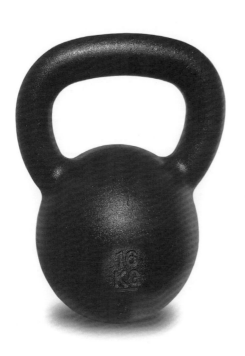
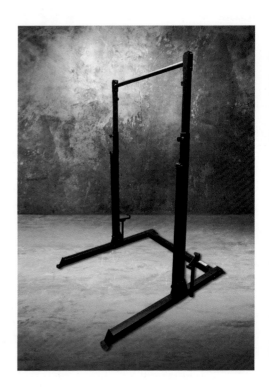

Trojan Framework for Group Sessions

	Time	Activity
	1-4 min.	Hip-stretch
		Shoulder rotations
	5-10 min.	Hardstyle plank: 10 sec. max effort
		Swing variations: 1- Deadlift 2- Double arm swing 3- Single arm swing
		Pushup variations: 1- From knees 2- Down from feet, up from knees 3- From hands and feet
Trojan Set:	11-19 min.	Plank — 10 sec. hardstyle plank
		Swing — 5-10 reps
		Push-ups — 3-10 reps
		Rest, repeat as many times as possible in 5 minutes
	20-24 min.	Lying leg-raise extension
		Kettlebell Squat variations 1. Goblet squat 2. Narrow squat 3. Pistol L/R
		Pull-up 1. Australian pull-up 2. Jump-pull up/ use dynaband 3. Strict pull-up
Trojan Set:	25-30 min.	Lying leg-raise extension (hold for 10 sec.)
		Kettlebell Squat — 5-10 reps
		Pull-up — 3-8 reps
		Rest, repeat as many times as possible in 5 minutes
End drill (optional)	1 min.	Hang top position (Australian) Pull-up

Session Timeline

Minutes	Exercise	
0-4	warm-up	squats, hip-flexion, shoulder rotation, etc.
5-10		plank, swing, push-ups
11-19		plank push-ups
20-24		lying leg raise, kettlebell squat, pull-ups
25-30		lying leg raise, kettlebell squat, pull-ups

1. Warm-ups are done quickly and efficiently for 4-5 minutes; loose, warm, ready
2. Planks, Trojan Pose and other isometrics are hard-style; held for maximum 10 seconds
3. Swings are crisp, emphasizing hip snap
4. Push-ups are strict; emphasize the contraction of the abs
5. Lying leg raise extensions controlled; lower back stays on the ground
6. Kettlebell squats are deep, upright torso, vertical shins
7. Pull-ups are done with no knee kicking or contorting
8. Each exercise has three acceptable variations, based on ability
9. Often we end with 30-60 second static hold
10. Trojan Sets rotate 2-5 exercises, starting with an isometric contraction or hold

Exercise Intensity Amplifiers: easy to difficult exercise variants

Swing	Pushup	Kettlebell Squat	Pull-up
Deadlift	From knees	Goblet squat	Australian pull-up
Double arm swing	Down from feet, up from knees	Narrow squat	Jump-pull up/ use dynaband
Single arm swing		Pistol L/R	
	From hands and feet		Strict pull-up

GROUP LESSONS

When teaching the Trojan Workout to a group, everyone does the same generalized workout at the same time. What varies are the exercise variations. There are three variations for every movement and each creates varying intensities. The participants select one of three exercise variations, moderate, harder, hardest. What also varies are the reps. The goal is continual improvement for extended periods.

Regardless the initial level, the goal is improvement. Technique is critical. Regardless the exercise variation selected, the goal is to adhere to highly specific techniques. I insist participants use these techniques because they deliver optimal results. Sloppy technique results in injury. Better two perfect reps than twenty sloppy, potentially injurious reps.

The easiest way to acclimatize to the rigors of the Trojan Workout are to use (initially) the easiest exercise variation combined with low reps. Perfect the techniques, then in each subsequent session add reps. When reps exceed ten, drop the reps back down and try the "harder" exercise variation. Over time increase reps and eventually move on to the hardest technique associated with each core exercise.

Participants are free to rest as needed after a Trojan Set. Over time the trainee seeks to improve their work-to-rest rest ratio. Trojan Workout participants will all work together in the same timeframe using differing variations of the called-for exercise.

Trojan Workout participants take as much or as little time between sets on an as-needed basis. We push through every technique and work it hard. The individualized drills and intensities may vary but the overarching template stays the same.

From a psychological perspective, the value of the group dynamic is incalculable. Training in front of other people automatically elevates performance. There is an exhilaration that comes from the positive energy generated by the group collective that has to be experienced to be appreciated.

TOOLS OF A TROJAN

Breathing is an important part of the Trojan workout. My earliest experiences with regulated breath control came as a teenage karate fighter. You learn how to contract when being punched and you learn that your own punching power is amplified when a violent punch or kick is synchronized with an equally violent exhalation.

Combat breathing was taught in the special forces. Soldiers were taught to consciously take control of their breathing and with concentrated effort lower the rate of respiration. Combat breathing had a multitude of benefits. Done right, you would and could lower your heart rate through breath control, a wonderful attribute for someone in a life-threatening situation. The degree of mental control required to lower respiration has the additional benefit of taking the soldier's mind off doubt, second thoughts and fear.

Recovery breathing is different. I trained so much and so often that I got a lot of practice at becoming better at breathing. Over time my breathing technique evolved. I now strive for passive inhalation; I avoid gulping and forced inhalation. By being a passive breather, recovery occurs quicker. This takes discipline and practice. The better your breathing the quicker your recovery. Breathing should be naturally and harmoniously synchronized with the effort: we inhale on the eccentric and exhale on the concentric portion of every rep.

Recovery breathing has another advantage. If your muscles use more energy than is available, oxygen debt occurs. There is always enough oxygen in the body. What we do not have is the compound hemoglobin. Focus on breathing *out* rather than on breathing *in* between rounds of the Trojan Workout. This breathing tactic will help you recover much faster. Hyperventilating prevents adequate gas exchange from taking place in your lungs and your blood loses carbon dioxide because you're taking in oxygen at an unusually fast rate.

Power breathing is designed to maximize muscle tension. Muscle tension creates stability and enables the athlete to generate maximum strength. Power breathing is used in the Trojan Pose and all types and kinds of isometric holds. Power breathing is diaphragm breathing and is accomplished by beginning the breath in the stomach: expand the stomach in every direction, then the lungs. This is tension and expansion.

Breathe in deeply, from the pit of the stomach upward. On the exhalation, press your tongue to the roof of the mouth and exhale with a sharp hiss. Do this while contracting the centerline muscles. Use power breathing during an isometric hold. Use power breathing to extend a ten second plank. We use power breathing during the isometric holds that follow an explosive movement, like pressing a heavy kettlebell overhead.

Ratings

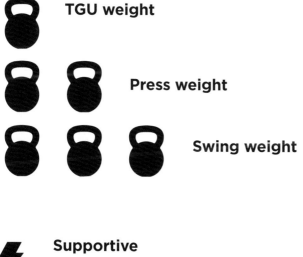

TGU weight

Press weight

Swing weight

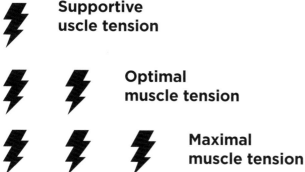

Supportive uscle tension

Optimal muscle tension

Maximal muscle tension

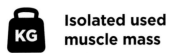 Isolated used muscle mass

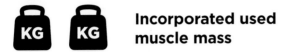 Incorporated used muscle mass

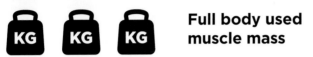 Full body used muscle mass

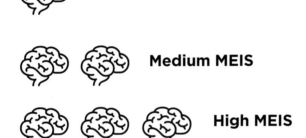

Low MEIS

Medium MEIS

High MEIS

Note; these are indications. Personal preferences and different body types can vary the rations per individual

ISOMETRIC HOLDS: THE TROJAN POSE

"You must commit to the contraction."

We consider isometric holds as a valuable part of every Trojan Workout. There is one special isometric hold that is the King exercise in every Trojan Workout: It's called the Trojan Pose.

- Start by standing tall
- Face forward and begin checking your posture
- Bare feet are connected to the surface you are standing on
- Legs are straight
- The spine is upright
- Shoulder are not sagging forward
- Tension in the abs
- Shoulder blades point to your opposite hipbones
- Neck straight and chin tucked

Check and adjust the posture: this is an awareness exercise; now increase isometric muscle tension

- Toes: dig them into the ground like they are claws
- Knees: lock them, increase tension around kneecaps
- Feet: screw your feet into the ground
- Squeeze the adductor muscles
- Squeeze the glutes
- Squeeze the abs
- Pull the shoulder blades inwards and down
- Squeeze the abs even more
- Lock the elbows
- Squeeze hands into fists

- Pull your chin in
- Breathe out using the Power Breathing 'hiss'
- Tense all muscles at the same time
- Create perfect posture
- The Trojan Pose never lasts more than ten seconds

Perfecting the Trojan Pose requires focus and practice. While performing the Trojan Pose, scan the body: where can you add more tension? An additional benefit: doing Trojan pose on a regular basis teaches the tension required in the ending position of the basic exercises: squat, push-up, pull-up, press, kettlebell swing, Turkish getup...all the end positions are locked in with full tension, like the Trojan Pose. Practice makes perfect!

Trojan Pose
1. Glutes **2.** Abs **3.** Quads **4.** Lats

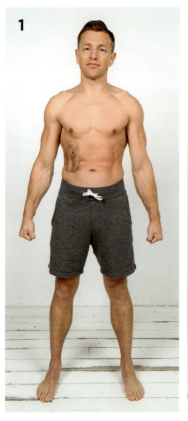
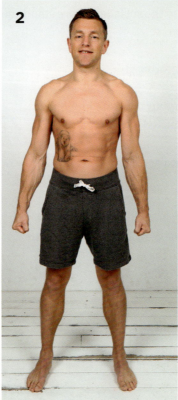
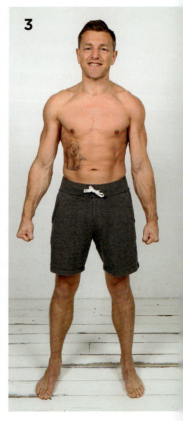

4

Key technical points: creating muscular tension is a learned skill. The greater the ability to tense the greater the hypertrophy and strength benefits: the four photos show ever-increasing degrees of tension.

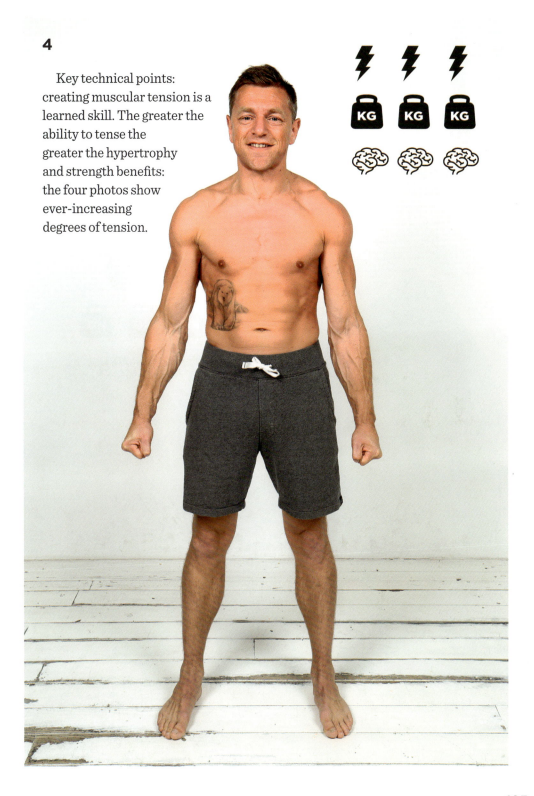

EXERCISES

Lunge

Key technical points: optimally the rear knee touches the floor on each and every step/rep. Strive for balance and seek to eliminate wobble. Play with stance width and always synchronize the stepping with breathing.

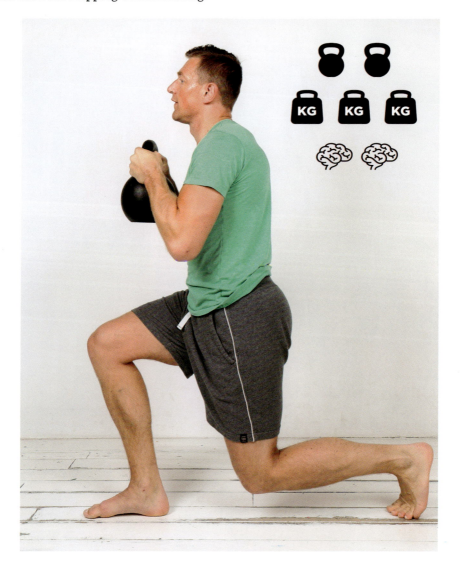

Jump up from Knees

Key technical points: this is an advanced exercise that not everyone can do. It requires coordination, timing and above all else explosiveness. at the top of the rep, kneel down to commence the next jump up rep.

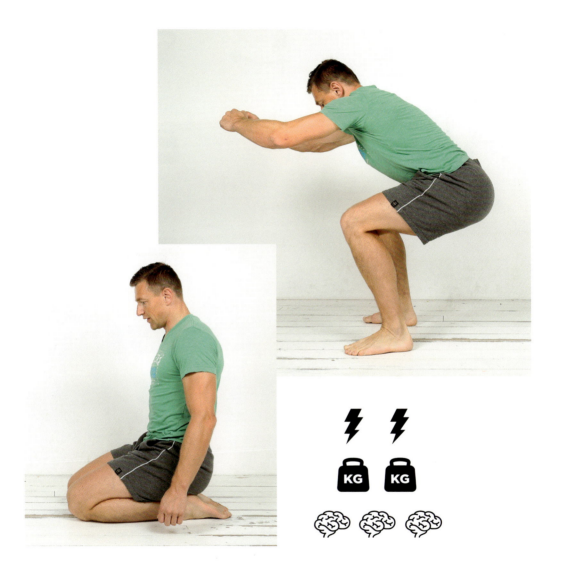

Kettlebell Swing

Key technical points: snap the hips forward at the apogee. Every rep need be crisp and distinctive. Exhale powerfully and audibly. The final position is the isometric Trojan pose.

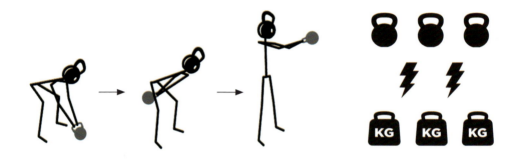

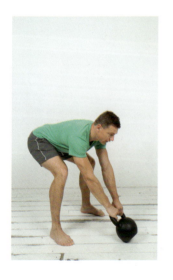

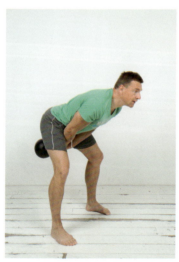

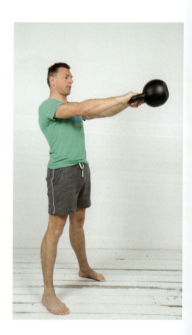

Thruster

Key technical points: every thruster begins with a full squat and is followed by a strict one arm press. Attention should be paid to balanced application: each side should be worked separately but equally.

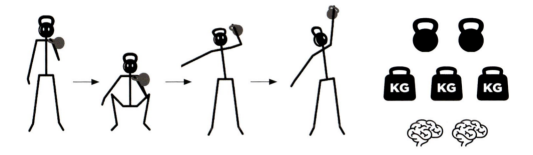

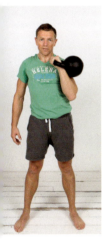 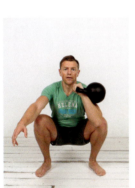 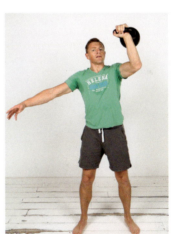 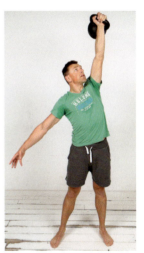

Stiff-leg Deadlift

Key technical points: the kettlebell is broken from the floor by activating the hip-hinge. The weight is lifted with straight arms and a rigid torso. The kettlebell is lifted and lowered using back power alone.

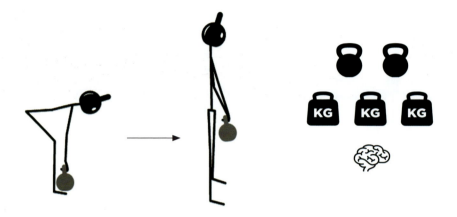

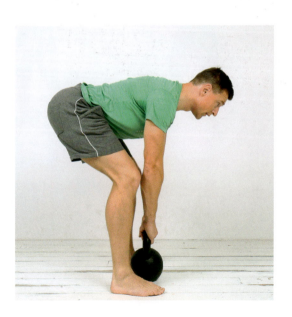

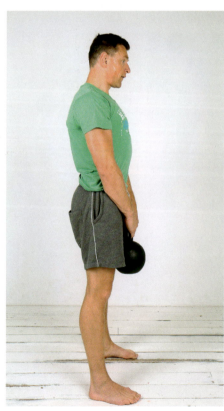

Horizontal Leg Extension

Key technical points: the goal is to generate a complete abdominal contraction on every repetitio. This is a 'continual tension' exercise. The motion needs to be complete and full on every repetition.

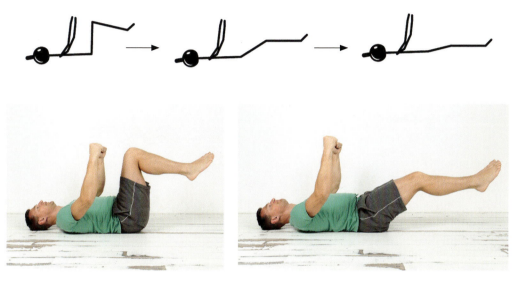

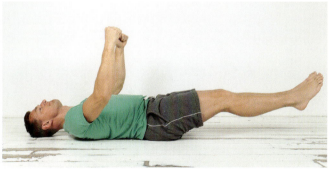

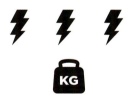

Lying Heel Press

Key technical point: the goal is to generate contraction in the glutes and posterior chain. The degree of contraction is determined by the tension generated from pressing the heels together while lifting the knees.

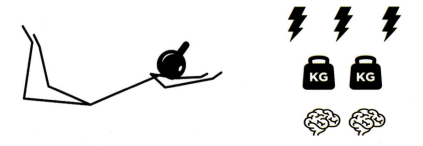

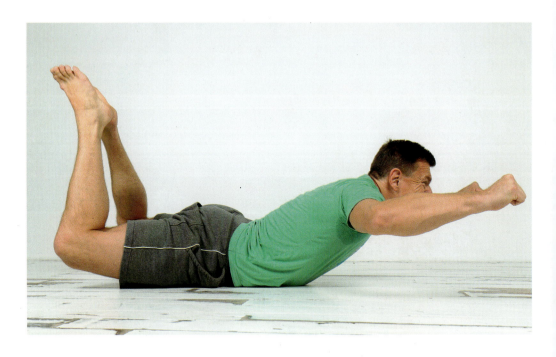

Sit and Reach Push

Key technical point: tension is generated using the hands to press thru the floor while lifting the legs. The raising of the legs creates incredible tension in the mid-section and can be modulated to a dramatic degree.

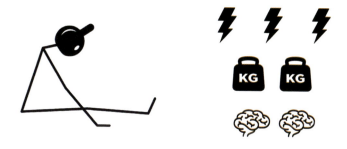

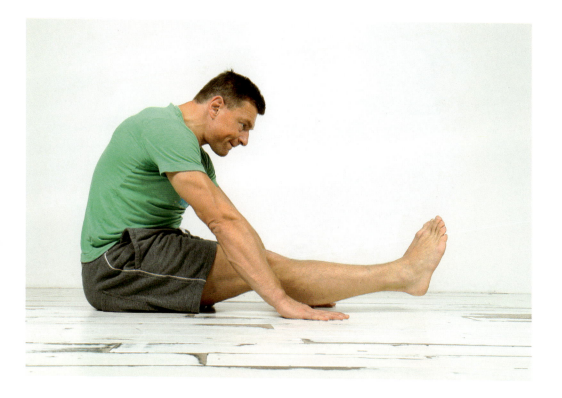

Cup Hold Bottom Squat

Key technical points: perhaps the most beneficial of all leg exercises is the goblet squat. Want to make a goblet squat much harder? Hold the payload out and in front of your eyes while squatting.

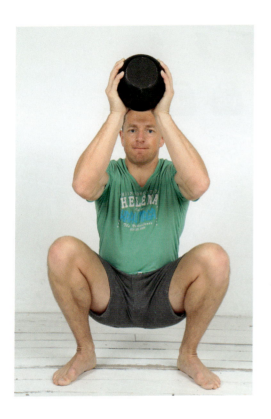
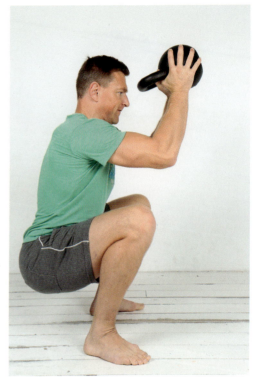

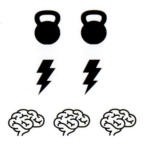

Trojan Pose Kettlebell Hold

Key technical points: this is a bold variation on the core Trojan Pose. The key to the Trojan Pose is the ability to create tension. For Trojan Pose adepts, amp up the intensity by holding a kettlebell at arms-length.

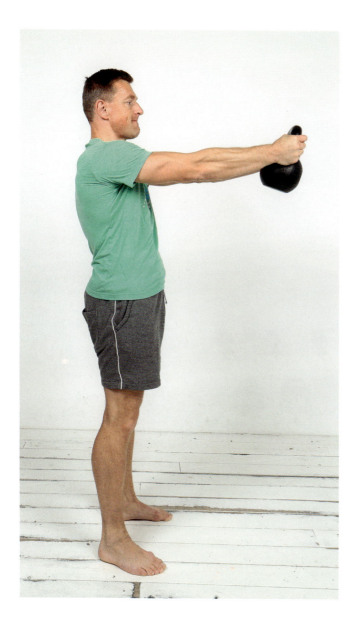

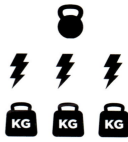

Plank

Key technical points: our planks don't sag. The perfect plank is another exercise is controlled tension. The harder you pull your elbows towards your toes, the greater the degree of tension generated.

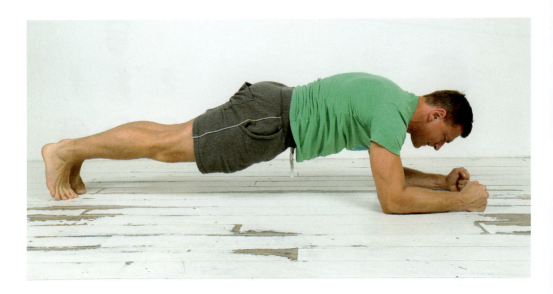

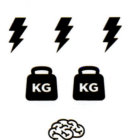

High Plank

Key technical points: the high plank creates stresses in completely different body regions. Increase the tension by pressing your toes thru the ground. Do not lose the pulling motion from palms to toes.

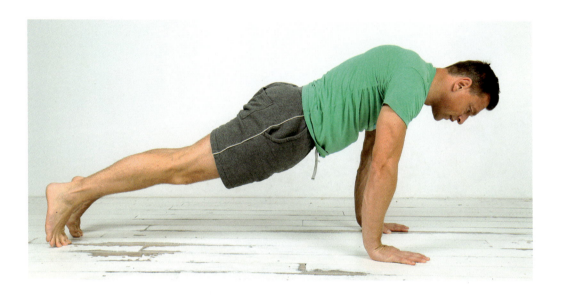

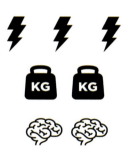

Knee to Elbow Isometric

Key technical points: tension done right builds power, strength and muscular endurance. You must commit to the contraction. Each side should receive equal doses of this superb exercise. Squeeze harder!

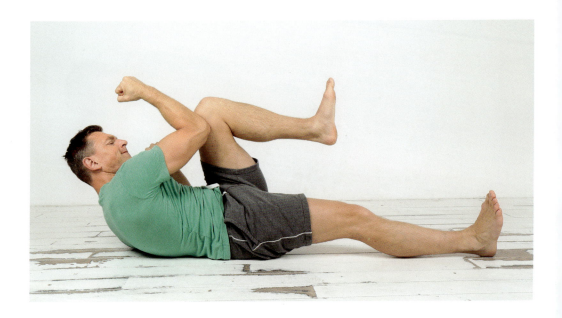

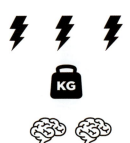

Quad Hold

Key technical points: how best to build and strengthen the powerful thigh muscles? The quad hold induces all the thigh tension a trainee can handle: to increase the severity, increase the angle and length of hold.

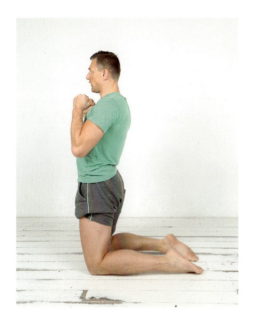
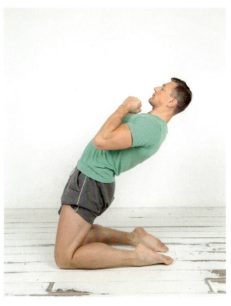
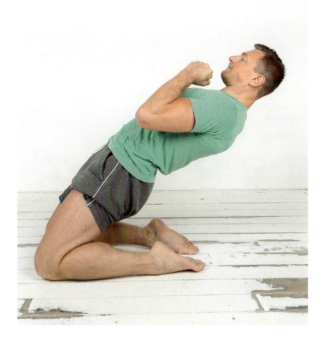
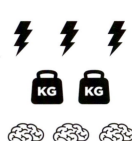

Lying Hip Thruster

Key technical points: full range-of-motion is critical in this unique movement. There are few activities in life that enable the athlete to drive the hip joint forward. Positioning is critical and technique is paramount.

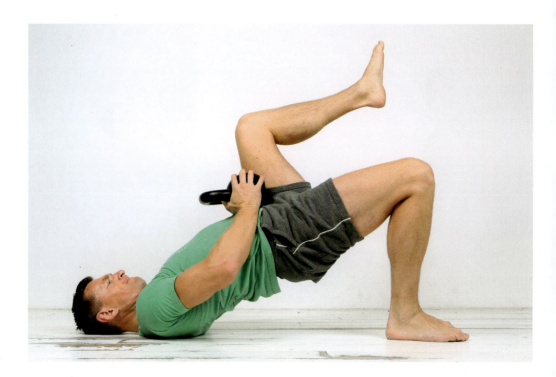

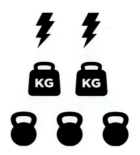

Lying Thruster Kettlebell Held Overhead

Key technical points: this variation uses a kettlebell to amplify the effects. The unique positioning of the arms creates a tension that needs to be experienced to the be believed. This is an advanced move.

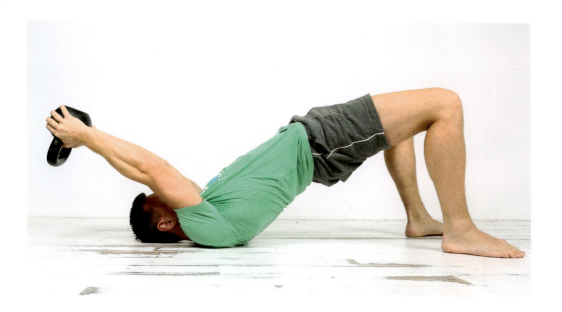

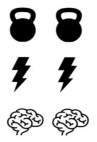

Wall Squat

Key technical points: the wall squat is the key to learning proper squat technique. The wall squat requires the knees be held over the ankles and the torso remain upright. This is the proper way to 'load' the thighs.

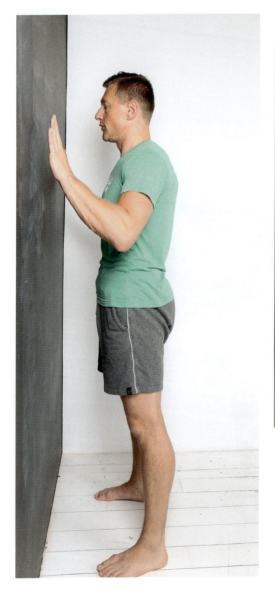

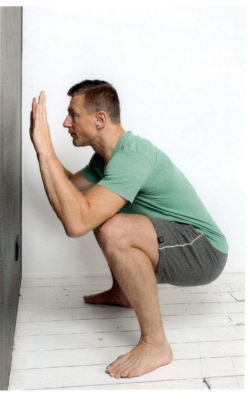

Kettlebell Goblet Squat

Key technical points: this squat variation is the King of leg exercises. No other single leg exercise stimulates the legs to the degree that a proper goblet squat does. Learn this key core exercise and master it.

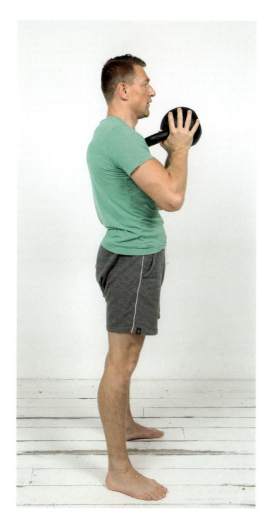
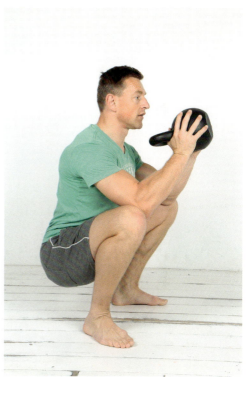
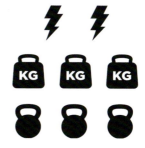

Narrow Squat

Key technical points: an excellent squat variation for the basic squat. The key is attaining full depth while keeping your knees glued together. Shallows squats deliver substandard results.

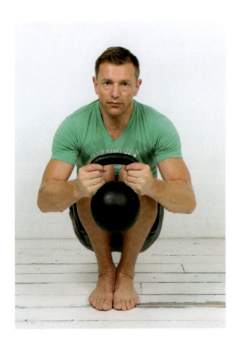
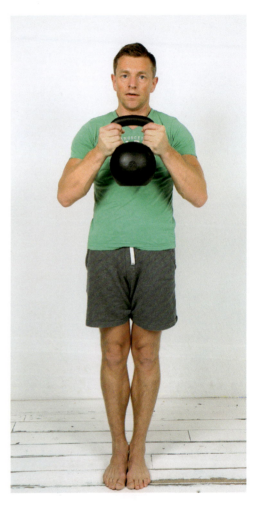
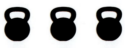

Horizontal Jumps

Key technical points: also known as standing broad jumps, repeated practice of high velocity leaping improves muscle tone, muscle strength and explosive power. Practice makes perfect with horizontal leaping.

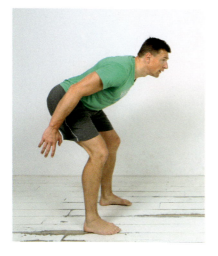
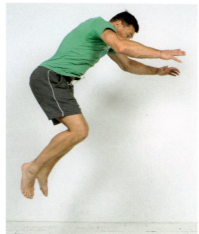
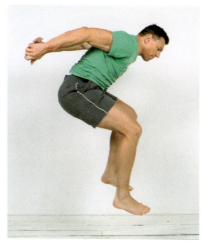
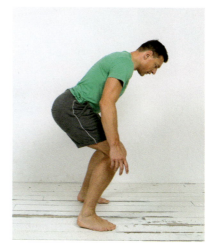

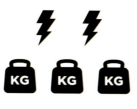

Overhead Press

Key technical points: this is a core strength movement. What is more natural in life than pushing a weight overhead. It is critical that there is an evenness and balance between your left and right arms.

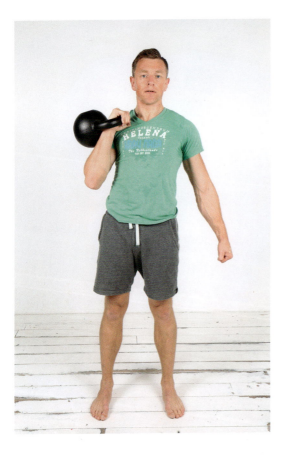

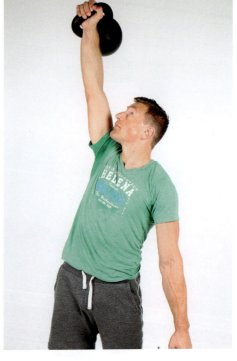

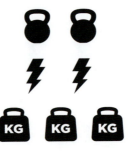

Lying Press

Key technical points: contract your core as hard as you can while pressing up. The lying press is a strong pushing position and allows the athlete to push maximum poundage and develop max power.

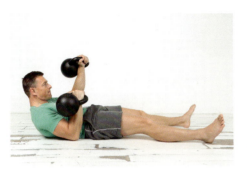
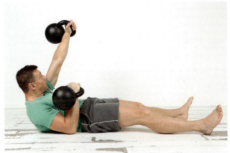
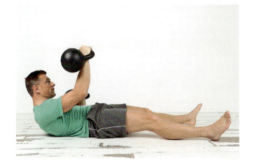
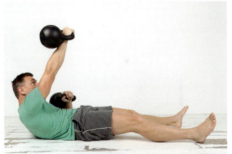

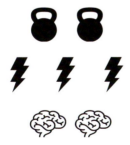

Car Wash

Key technical points: this is a continuous tension exercise that causes the shoulders to tremble and shake. The idea is to plank with one side while sliding up and down the opposite arm. A towel is optional.

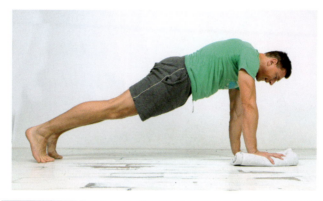

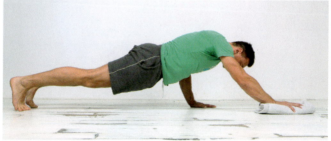

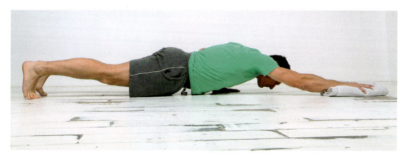

Mule Kick

Key technical points: maximum explosive leverage. The idea is to establish an ideal position from which to fire a maximum velocity rearward kick – maximum power with maximum velocity.

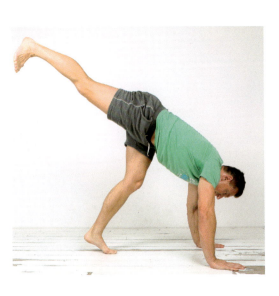
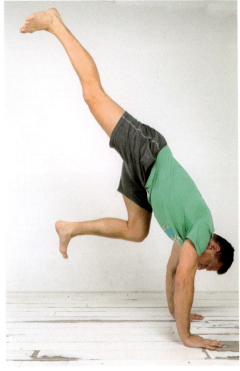
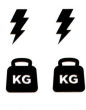

Full Mule Kick

Key technical points: while the Mule Kick is a single leg exercise – one leg then the other; the Full Mule Kick is when the athlete fires both legs simultaneously. The earmarks for both are velocity and power.

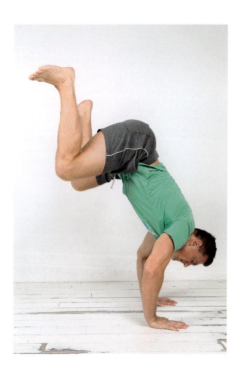 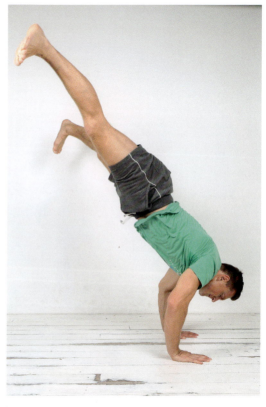

Push-up from Knees

Key technical points: the push-up done right is the ideal chest, arm and shoulder-strengthening exercise. The push-up done on the knees reduces the amount of bodyweight needing to be pushed. Strict form is critical.

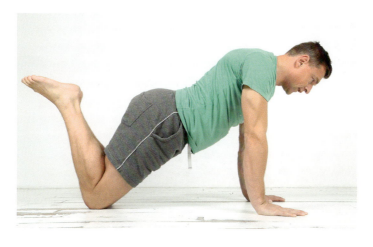

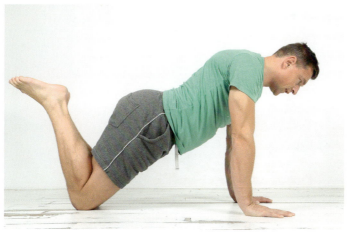

Push-up

Key technical points: the classical push-up requires strict form and technical perfection. Master the pushup off knees first. Graduate to the strict push-up: lower and raise holding a perfect plank.

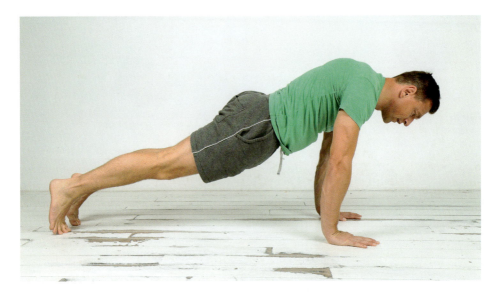

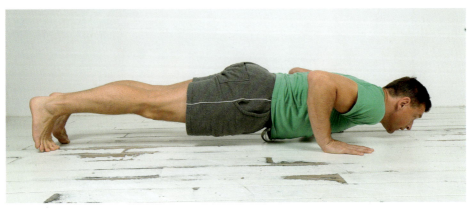

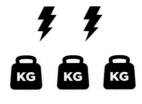

Turkish Get-up

Key technical points: this is a complex movement that requires complete attention to detail. Note the relationship of the kettlebell to the torso in each of the five photos. This exercise is unrivalled for creating stability.

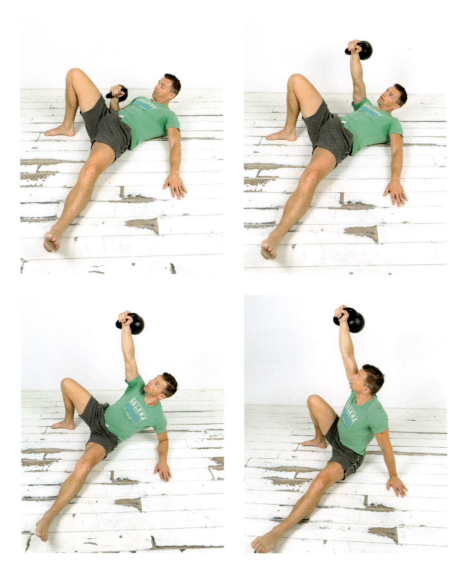

CONTINUED NEXT PAGE...

Turkish Get-up (continued)

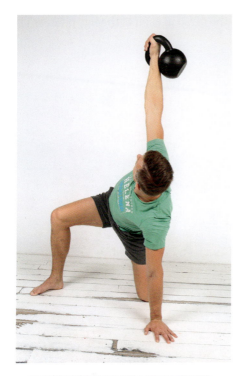
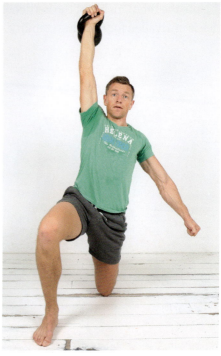
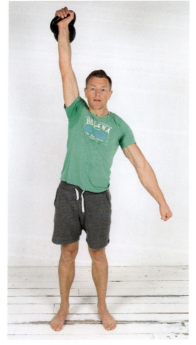
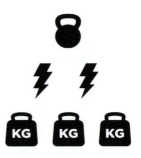

TROJAN SETS

- Pick an *isometric* exercise from column 1
- Pick a *ballistic* exercise from column 2
- Pick an *fast-paced* exercise from column 3
- Or choose an entire row

Isometric	Ballistic	Paced/ Grind
High Plank	Swing	TGU
Hardstyle Plank	Horizontal Jump	Push-up
Lying Heel Press	Thruster	Carwash
Lying hip thruster + kb OH	Alternating Lunge	Wall Ssquat
Cup Hold	Narrow Squat	Press
Trojan Pose	Swing-step Forward 10m	Drag back swing 10 m
Cup Hold	Squat	Lunge Position Press
TP hold + kb	Squat	Walk 10-20m with kb Forward
Quad hold from Kneeling	jump up from Knees	Archer Push-up
Hardstyle Plank	Press	SCDL – Farmer Walk
Lying Press	Lunge + Rotate kb Front Leg	Ab rotation from Kneeling
horizontal Leg Extension	Mule Kick	Lying Press
Bottom Squat Cup Hold	Stop Swing – Horizontal Jump (ladder 1-10)	Push-up
Sit and Reach Push	Deadlift	Bear Crawl
Knee to Elbow Hold	SL lying bridge	Push-up kb Drag

You will find additional information for this section and an easy-to-use app that guides you in your *Trojan Sets* at:

TRAINING TIPS WHEN TRAINING AT HOME (NO GROUP SESSION)

When doing Trojan Workout at home, beginners should perform one Trojan Set every minute. Beginners should start with a ten-minute session length. Each subsequent Trojan Workout training session, add one minute to the session length until 30-minute sessions are achieved. Aim for ten-second contractions in all isometric tension exercises. Select the appropriate number of your personal rep range (3-10 reps) for the ballistic and fast-paced exercises. For every exercise, you pick a variation. Keep the same numbers for every set.

You will find additional information about this section and for a guided workout at:

TROJAN WORKOUT FOR SELF-DEFENSE

I strongly believe that serious Krav Maga students need formalized strength training. Krav Maga teaches how to defend yourself. But without the ability to generate some strength and a minimum of muscle tension, your overall performance stays limited. A weakling can be overwhelmed, no matter how good their techniques. And strength is a skill that you need to learn.

As American boxer and puncher-supreme Mike Tyson once eloquently said, "All the plans and strategies go out the window once you get punched in the face." Indeed, then it becomes survival. I have been punched in the face many times. I have punched people in the face many times. As a result, I have a high pain tolerance that only comes from continual and ongoing exposure to pain. How else would you extend your pain capacity other than repeatedly experiencing it?

I wanted to address what I perceived as a chink in the psychological armor of my Krav Maga students. Combat martial arts should not be an academic exercise. Part of fighting is fighting. Fighters fight. Otherwise they are not fighters, they are hobbyists and voyeurs. You cannot understand the essence of combat fighting without experiencing all that goes with fighting someone way better than you. Or multiple attackers. Or people with weapons intent on harming you.

There is this myth that a magical system of self-defense exists that easily and effortlessly defends against the most savage of attacks. This is pure nonsense and can get you killed. Defending yourself is always *stressful* and never easy. To defend yourself you need to hurt the attacker. That is part of my job. My job as an Krav Maga instructor is (among other things) teaching people to hurt other people.

True self-defense, Krav Maga self-defense, requires you respond to aggression with aggression. Those that are trained, those that are ready, willing and able to defend themselves carry themselves with a certain self-confidence that reduces the likelihood of an attack. Human predators select the weakest prey as their victims.

An overlooked aspect of self-defense is conflict prevention. So many violent incidents would be eliminated if the victim exhibited the confidence that goes with deep knowledge of Krav Maga. Bad people will reconsider before bothering you. I teach this "mental stance" approach ("Stand strong in your shoes!") to my students.

A person can study a martial art and learn that this counter is the proper response, the counter move, selected like a thoughtful move in a chess match. You never have the time to sort through the multiple mental possibilities while the attacker is attacking. Krav Maga teaches intuitive response—the highest form of martial arts. Krav Maga and the Trojan Workout both stress the physical and the psychological. We combine knowledge with application.

How do you explain and demonstrate the idea of mental toughness? How do you explore and expand one's ability to hang out for extended periods in the discomfort and pain zone? How do you teach normal people to take initiative and actually attack another human being? I explain that it is for their own wellbeing.

This is usually when the person new to Krav Maga asks, "Isn't there a non-hurtful way to counter a predator's attack?" Again, this is an unrealistic belief. It can take some mental recalibration on the part of the student to grasp that, yes, to deal effectively with a predator's attack you are going to have to hurt them!

Fine and upstanding citizens do not visit violence on others. My strategy is to plainly explain why we were going to perform a particular drill in a particular way and then, as a group, we realistically workshop the technique—with as much realism, intensity and contact as the limits would allow.

We never seek to injure ourselves or our training partners, however it is the duty of every Krav Maga practitioner to seek realism and seek to exceed current capacities in every way, shape and form.

I always sought to devise drills that allowed trainees to push the limits of the envelope. Every training session represents an opportunity to improve some aspect of our Krav Maga. I began mentally formulating a companion physical training protocol, one specifically devised to improve skills and capabilities associated with high level Krav Maga.

What physical attributes could enhance the Krav Maga trainee's performance? I had spent my whole life training to become a better martial artist.

Eventually, you have to look outside the martial art to improve the martial art. Once all the techniques are learned, once all the releases, defenses and counters are explained and drilled, once you learn everything there is to know about a martial art, everything is now just rearranging the contents of the box: you need to step outside the box.

The way to improve as a martial artist is to do as Bruce Lee did and seek to build a better body. How does one define "better body?" In the case of Krav Maga, better body would be leaner (lower body fat), more powerful (more lean muscle mass), possessing superior endurance and an ability to generate sustained strength for extended periods.

The fitness training created for Krav Maga would be designed to make the athlete faster, more agile, with superior stamina and strength, a higher pain tolerance and an open and alert mind, ready to spontaneously react in an appropriate manner to threats as they spontaneously arise. Trojan Workout is the answer.

What type of drills could be used to improve the physical body of the Krav Maga trainee? I was my own ongoing lab experiment. I tried out all my strategies on myself and on my students. What better way to test the effectiveness of a strategy than to test it myself?

KRAV MAGA IN MOTION

Basic drills for awareness

One of the many aspects of Krav Maga that separates it from other martial arts is the Krav Maga emphasis on what in Spec Ops is called, "situational awareness." What is the situation you are in currently? In Krav Maga a "360-degree arc of awareness" is taught. Situational awareness is a learned skill. Awareness drills are a big part of the Krav Magaphilosophy. Here are some drills and variations we use to teach awareness.

- In the dojo or training studio the drill calls for all the Krav Maga students to commence running around the room, changing direction every 5-6 steps. During this milling about, I yell, "BLUE!" and now everyone scrambles to seize a blue object or touch a blue color.

- A variation on this basic milling about in nonchalant fashion: I yell, "DOOR!" and every student now scrambles to exit the nearest door. Often in the door drill students run into each other rushing through doorways. This is workshopped.

- The third variation on the crowd scenario is everyone is running around when I yell "WEAPON!" An appropriate response to weapon would be to grab a common object for your own weapon.

- The response for "GUN!" might be to run out the nearest door.

- Divide a few training knives among the group. While running across the room, students keep passing the knife to another student. When I give a signal (no one knows who has the knives) the students that are holding the knives attack the other students.

- With children: I hide a knife somewhere in the room. The kids try to find it as soon as possible. The one who finds it, raises it up in the air. The others need to point to the knife, warn the others by screaming and run to the door immediately.

- Make pairs: one partner holds a punching shield. Everyone runs around in the training area. On my count, the ones with the punching shield stands still, the other partner needs to find and attack the shield holder as soon as possible.

- To find the partner that is holding the pad, you need to scan the area. Then, as soon as you see him/her, you need to turn into aggressor mode, run as fast as possible to the pad and attack it at full speed and power.

Once you understand the principles of Trojan Workout and the concept of the Trojan sets, you can, as a kravist use this knowledge for combining Trojan Workout with Krav Maga skill training.

Below you find some Trojan Set examples combined with Krav Maga skills. According to your Krav Maga level, you can use these sets for training under (physical) stress while improving your overall Krav Maga performances as well as your strength, speed and stamina.

Isometric	Ballistic	Paced	Level
Knee to Elbow Hold	KM Getup	Push Walk 10-20m	P1
High elbow Palm Push-pull	ChokeReleases	Floor Elbow Drag	P1
OA Pushing Hold	Straight Cross Punch	Under hook control partner	P1
Hardstyle Plank	Elbow Strikes	Fighting from clinch	P1
Pull-up Hold	Bridge up from Bottom Position Mounth	Trying to get up against pads holding you down	P2
High March Hold	High Kicks	Squats	P2
Spider Hold	Hook Punches	Fighting for Underhooks	P2
Push against pad/ Partner	Punching Combos	Bearhug Lifting	P3
High Plank	Scissors Kicks	Passing Crowd	P4
Hold Partner	Breakfall	Fighting from Guard	P5
Press Elbow on Knee in Guard	Kick up	Grapple for Position	G1
Wall Push Legs	Vertical jump/Swing	Takedowns	G2

You will find additional information for this section and highly effective Trojan Sets for Krav Maga at: